PRAISE FOR *SUBU*
TALES I
MEDICINE'S I

'Cecil Helman is many things: old-fashioned general practitioner, psychiatrist, cultural anthropologist, storyteller, poet and artist – and all of this comes together in *Suburban Shaman*, a beautifully written, devastatingly honest (and often very funny) account of an audacious and adventurous life.'

Oliver Sacks
Neurologist and author of *The Man Who Mistook His Wife for a Hat, Awakenings* and *Hallucinations*

'I simply could not put down this extraordinary mixture of stories from the GP's surgery in suburban London ... Two clear messages emerge from this book, which should be required reading for every medical student ... First, medicine must relearn its heart and soul ... Second, there is no certainty in medicine, and no clear answer as to what it is that cures, or fails to cure people ... Clearly told, and an extraordinary read, this is a passionate cry for humane medicine.'

Rabbi Julia Neuberger, the Baroness Neuberger DBE
Senior Rabbi, Member of the House of Lords, Writer
The Independent

'A marvellous memoir on the human side of GP practice ... His resolutely non-specialist memoir may, I think, turn out to be one of the classics which every medical student *must* read ... I don't think anyone since AJ Cronin has expressed so strongly what it is to be embedded in the community as a GP.'

Libby Purves OBE
Presenter, journalist and author
BBC Radio 4 *Midweek*

ALSO BY THE AUTHOR

Culture, Health & Illness, 5th edition
(2009)

Suburban Shaman: Tales from Medicine's Frontline
(2006)

Doctors and Patients: an Anthology
(2002)

The Body of Frankenstein's Monster: Essays in Myth and Medicine
(1992)

Body Myths
(1991)

The Golden Toenails of Ambrosio P
(1990)

Prose poems

Irregular Numbers of Beasts and Birds
(2006)

The Girl on the Aeroplane
(2002)

The Exploding Newspaper and Other Fables
(1981)

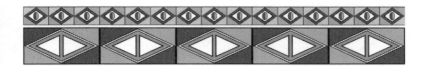

AN AMAZING MURMUR OF THE HEART

FEELING THE PATIENT'S BEAT

CECIL HELMAN

Hammersmith Health Books
London, UK

First published in 2014 by Hammersmith Health Books – an imprint of Hammersmith Books Limited
14 Greville Street, London EC1N 8SB, UK
www.hammersmithbooks.co.uk

Author's note
Where the Author has included case histories, descriptions of patients, or dialogue, usually recreated from memory after many years or even decades, he has taken considerable care in each case to protect the identity of the people involved. He has changed a variety of medical, personal, historical and other identifying details, including sometimes the time, place and circumstances of the encounter – in some cases blending similar stories together. Despite this occasional but very necessary 'fictionalisation' to protect identity, every single one of the case histories is based originally on real people and on real events. The Author was very grateful to the people concerned, and hoped he described them with the respect and compassion that they deserve. He was also confident that anyone who thinks they recognise themselves in a case history will be mistaken, for he has deliberately selected stories that are in some ways archetypal, with each one representing many hundreds of very similar cases that would be familiar to any family doctor, in almost every practice in the land.

British Library Cataloguing in Publication Data: A CIP record of this book is available from the British Library.

ISBN (print edition): 978-1-78161-019-0
ISBN (ebook): 978-1-78161-020-6

Commissioning editor: Georgina Bentliff
Designed and typeset by: Julie Bennett, Bespoke Publishing Ltd
Production by: Helen Whitehorn, Path Projects Ltd
Printed and bound by: TJ International Ltd, UK
Cover illustration by: Christopher Hoare

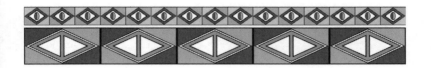

CONTENTS

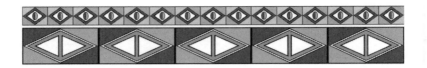

PUBLISHER'S NOTE

It was a great honour for Hammersmith Press to publish Cecil Helman's *Suburban Shaman* in 2006. With the help of publicist Pam Solomon, it was widely and positively reviewed and read on BBC Radio 4 as *Book of the Week*.

Even before it was published, Cecil was working on this second collection of medical stories and the general issues about medical practice and contemporary medical training that they prompted. He read from both collections at literary events between 2006 and 2009, but increasingly he had to ask others to read for him as his throat was giving him trouble – the first signs of the motor neurone disease that was eventually to kill him.

Cecil died in June 2009 just as retirement from research and teaching was offering the opportunity to write full time. This was a great loss to us all. Thankfully he entrusted *An Amazing Murmur of the Heart*, his final manuscript, to his daughter Zoe, and his close friends Clive Sinclair and Doron Swade. Hammersmith Books is now delighted to publish it as both a print and an ebook – an option that was only in its infancy when Cecil died. These stories remind us of Cecil's humanity as a doctor and his erudition and breadth of vision as a writer – aspects of himself that he would hope to pass on to all who read his last book.

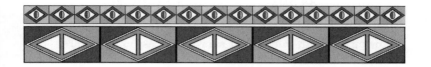

ABOUT CECIL HELMAN

Dr Cecil Helman was born in Cape Town, South Africa, into a family of doctors and artists. He studied medicine there during the apartheid era before moving to the UK, where he studied anthropology at University College London.

After a spell as a ship's doctor, he became a family practitioner in London while also developing a distinguished academic career, focusing on the cross-cultural study of health, illness and medical care – a specialism he largely established. He was a Visiting Fellow in Social Medicine and Health Policy at Harvard Medical School and a Visiting Professor in the Multi-cultural Health Programme at the University of New South Wales. He retired from clinical practice in 2002 but continued his academic work, being Professor of Medical Anthropology at Brunel University and Senior Lecturer in the Department of Primary Care & Population Sciences, Royal Free & University College Medical School, London, UK until his death in 2009. His leading textbook, *Culture, Health and Illness* is now in its fifth edition, published by CRC Press, and has been translated into many other languages.

In recognition of his pioneering achievements, Cecil received two major international awards for his work:

- the Career Achievement Award of the American Anthropological Association (2004), and
- the Lucy Mair Medal for Applied Anthropology of the Royal Anthropological Institute (2005).

In addition to his academic achievements, Cecil was a talented writer of stories, prose poems and essays. The autobiographical *Suburban Shaman* was published in 2009 to great acclaim. For it he won the Royal College of General Practitioners' Abercrombie Medal 'for an outstanding contribution to the literature of general practice' and the Book of the Year award from the Society of Medical Writers in 2007. *An Amazing Murmur of the Heart* is published posthumously, following his death from motor neurone disease in June 2009.

'Spending time with Cecil was like being in one of his books. He gave much thought and meaning to everyday experience and, always the enquiring and informed observer, would reveal his quizzical insights when one least expected it. [He] was a generous man, always helpful and encouraging of others' projects and growth.'

From Gerald Mars's obituary of Cecil Helman, *The Guardian*

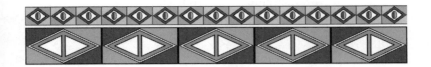

INTRODUCTION

'The practice of medicine is an art, based on science.'
Sir William Osler

This book is about healing and curing, and the differences between the two.

I have used the word 'healing' for the care of the ill person. As well as treating their symptoms, it means listening to the stories they tell, and dealing with their fears, hopes, dreams and desires. 'Curing', by contrast, focuses mainly on the care of the body itself, its diseases and dysfunctions, often at the level of its organs or cells.

Healing is about people; curing is about patients.

Many of the stories in *An Amazing Murmur of the Heart* – told from both sides of the doctor's desk – are about the widening gap between these two approaches in modern medicine, and the great distress this can cause. Most of them are based on my own experience – on the cases that I have observed, and the lessons I have learned, during 27 years as a family doctor in London and surrounding towns. But it also draws on my studies in social anthropology shortly after finishing medical school, combined with a long-term interest in mythology, folklore and traditional healing practices; and also on a research project I carried out at Harvard Medical School in the 1980s.

The stories included here deal mainly with the *non*-medical aspects of illness and of medical care. They show how different people respond in very different ways to suffering and illness. This more personal, intimate perspective is one that you will rarely find described in any conventional medical textbook, with its 'one-size-fits-all' approach to medical treatment. And yet understanding each person's unique responses to illness is crucial for successfully healing them, as well as curing their ailing bodies. This is something that every patient knows – and every doctor should.

In the Introduction to his classic *Cambridge Illustrated History of Medicine*, the historian Roy Porter points out a key paradox at the heart of modern medicine: 'Never have people in the West lived so long, or been so healthy, and never have medical achievements been so great. Yet, paradoxically, rarely has medicine drawn such intense doubts and disapproval as today.'

This odd situation is something I've puzzled over for very many years, both before and after I entered practice. While doctors are as committed as they ever were to the relief of human suffering, why is it that every year there is an increasing number of complaints against them? Why the rising rates of litigation? Why the media campaigns that publicise medicine's failings, often more than its successes? And why are more and more people resorting to 'alternative' types of health care, instead of its conventional forms? Is it just due to the growth of a more educated, perhaps more demanding, patient population, with over-inflated expectations of what medicine can actually deliver? Or is it maybe a reaction to a certain direction in which medicine itself is developing?

In answering these questions, any criticism of medicine always has to be balanced with an acknowledgement of all its many triumphs, especially in the Western world over the past century or so. Some have resulted from better public health measures, others from specific medical breakthroughs. There has been a dramatic decline in infant mortality (in Britain, a drop from 140 deaths per 1000 live births in 1900, to only 5.6 in 2000); the decline in maternal mortality, both during and after childbirth; the increase in life expectancy; and the development of new vaccines that have virtually eradicated many diseases – such as smallpox, polio, diphtheria, typhoid and measles – once the scourge of previous generations. Other medical discoveries have produced new and effective drugs to fight infection, improve cardiac function, relieve pain, and help contain terrible diseases such as malaria and tuberculosis. Developments in 'spare part surgery' have made a wide range of transplants and prostheses available to replace organs or body parts, once they have become damaged or worn out. Diagnostic technology now enables doctors to precisely identify the presence of severe diseases, even at a very early stage. And *in vitro* fertilisation (IVF) and surrogate pregnancy both offer new hope for infertile women.

Despite this, some critics prefer to focus on well-publicised medical disasters, such as the thalidomide tragedy, the increasing side-effects of many drugs and other treatments, and the contamination of transfused blood by the HIV virus – all of which have helped undermine public trust in the medical profession. There is also the growing cost of medical care and medical bureaucracy, and the rushed and pressurised consultations, long-waiting lists, and sometimes impersonal, mass-produced approach of the National Health Service. For many people, though, the dissatisfaction seems to be with a type of medicine that focuses only on a fragment of a body, rather than on the whole person. A mostly technical, mechanistic approach that tends to treat specific diseases – rather than the people who have those diseases.

My own particular background, from childhood onwards, prepared me for a very different approach to medicine – a long-term interest in its less technical, more holistic aspects. I grew up in South Africa in a family that produced a dozen doctors, and many other relatives who also worked in the health field, as medical social workers, medical librarians, or laboratory technicians. Listening to my father, a consultant psychiatrist, and my uncles and cousins telling their tales to one another about the unusual cases they'd just encountered, the diagnoses that they'd made or missed, all made it clear to me early on that medicine was a literary, as well as a technical, discipline. It was not just about science – it was also all about *stories* – the stories that sick people tell themselves, and their doctors, about why they got ill in the first place. And it's about how those narratives then mingle with those of the doctor during the medical consultation.

In addition, two of my uncles – one an eminent gastroenterologist, the other a paediatrician – shared a special interest in the 'psychosomatic' approach to medicine. Their aim was not only to treat bodily diseases, but also to understand the complex links between body and mind that accompany them. Doctors of that generation, in the infancy of the great technological breakthroughs that have transformed medical diagnosis, well understood that physical disease is never just a physical phenomenon and that it could never really be understood if viewed only through a scientific or a statistical lens, or somehow separated from the rest of that individual's life. Disease was always accompanied by less tangible elements, such as its emotional or social impact, or the role of the context in which it occurred.

I suspect that they would be envious of, but also baffled by, the emergence of a new type of doctor – the one I call the 'techno-doctor'. This highly skilled individual is often someone with an overriding obsession with technology, and usually a super-specialist with an interest in only a small area of the body. A doctor who sees the body merely as a repairable machine, rather than as part of a suffering person – a machine that can best be diagnosed, and then treated, only by other machines. Or merely as a complex assemblage of cells, enzymes, sinews and bones, and not much more than that. As a result they tend to over-emphasise the physical aspects of illness while dismissing as largely irrelevant its wider emotional, social, cultural and even spiritual dimensions. Their focus is almost exclusively on phenomena located *within* the body – arteries that clog up, cells that proliferate too wildly, joints that wear away, or glands that produce too little or too much of a particular hormone – while largely ignoring the impact of these events on the rest of the patient's world: their personal lives; their relationships with others; their jobs, housing or love life; or even their religious beliefs.

They are the doctors who have elevated the Science of medicine, way above its Art.

One day, early in the Cape summer, sometime towards the end of 1967, a friend and I are roaming the wards of Groote Schuur Hospital, our university teaching hospital, looking for 'interesting cases' to examine. It is only a few weeks before our final medical school exams, and we are frantically trying to examine as many patients as possible while we can, to improve our clinical skills – to listen to their wheezing chests, palpate their swollen abdomens, probe into this orifice or that. In every other ward of the teaching hospital, hordes of other white-coated medical students are also busy on the same frantic journey. Everyone is tense.

In one of the medical wards we are sent by one of the junior doctors to examine an elderly man, pale and wheezing in his bed. He is courteous and cooperative, but we are soon bored by his story, and by the 'physical signs' revealed by our examination. We grumble to the ward doctor afterwards that it's 'just another case of heart failure'. Nothing special. We've seen dozens of them already in the past few months, and why has he wasted our time on something so common, so ordinary?

The doctor doesn't say anything, but there's a strange look in his eye. And just a short time later, at the end of that year, we learn the reason why. For that elderly man has become the recipient of the world's first heart transplant, one of the greatest milestones in medical history. His face is now one of the most famous in the world, featured in every newspaper, glowing on every television screen. He is more famous than any of us will ever be. And what's more, the heart surgeon Dr Christiaan Barnard is one of our own lecturers.

And yet, even at the time, I was convinced that all this enormous worldwide attention couldn't possibly be due only to the daring, technical brilliance of the operation. Something else has happened, something much more significant that could not be explained only in strictly medical terms. For it is almost as if Dr Barnard had somehow strayed inadvertently into a landscape of signs and metaphors, where the word 'heart' referred not only to a small muscular pump inside the chest, but also stood as a universal symbol of emotion, intimacy, courage and will. For the first time in human history one of the most important metaphors for personhood had been cut out, handled, cleaned, and then placed inside the body of another individual. In just a few historic minutes, the borders of one human being had been breached by the symbolic core of another.

Long after the operation was over I found that those familiar idioms that I'd always used – such as 'to take heart', 'with all my heart', 'sick of heart' or 'to have one's heart in the right place' – had all acquired a peculiar new salience, a double meaning both medical and metaphorical. For during the transplant operation, the recipient was literally 'heartless' for those brief, but by now famous, moments as the surgeon lifted the old broken heart out of his body and handed it to an assistant – before replacing it inside the empty chest with the healthier heart of another. In this way, the donor had literally 'given heart' to the recipient, while each had 'lost their heart' to the other via the matchmakers of surgical science.

I am sure that none of this was on Dr Barnard's mind during the operation as, with sharply focused attention, he cut and clamped and sewed, taking out one heart, putting in another. And yet this unique surgical operation seems to me to mark a significant watershed, a moment of convergence between the worlds of medicine and those of metaphor and myth. For one dizzying moment in 1967, the protective boundary between Nature and Art, between physical reality and the language that we use to signify it, was suddenly dissolved. And therefore I was not at all surprised some time later, to read in the newspaper how, after an American patient had received the world's first artificial heart – a clever little device of steel, rubber and plastic – his wife was quoted as saying how relieved she was to find that he still loved her, and the children as well.

Perhaps for the first time in my medical career I came to realise how the human body was much more than a physical object, which was sometimes healthy and sometimes ill. It is always much more than that. Unlike its portrayal in the medical textbooks, the body also has powerful symbolic and cultural meanings. It is always linked intimately to language, metaphor and idiom. And sick people always live within a much larger picture – whether social, cultural, or economic – that can shape their experience of bodily illness and how it is treated. It is a lesson that I have never forgotten.

And yet, at medical school no-one ever taught us about the possible role of metaphor and myth in influencing how patients interpret their symptoms. Nobody described in any detail to us how patients' belief systems, or their cultural background, could either damage or improve their health. Nobody ever mentioned the theatrical side of medical care – how illness could be presented, not in words but by an intricate dance of symptoms, a mime of movements and facial expressions, that might take months or even years to display – and even longer for the doctor to decode. And therefore, how time and patience were so crucial for patient care. No-one described to us with any clarity the role of the inner worlds of doctor and patient, and how the doctor's own emotions could influence his or her reactions to different types of patients. My colleagues and I have all had to fill in these gaps ourselves, from our own studies, and from our own clinical experiences, over the years.

An Amazing Murmur of the Heart is a further attempt to explain the gaps between healing and curing, by illustrating that you cannot ever understand medical practice – and why it works or doesn't work – from a purely scientific perspective. For so much more is happening than ever meets the eye – hidden dimensions that simply cannot be scanned or X-rayed, or even described adequately in a medical textbook. To truly understand them one needs to delve deeper into the symbols and myths that people use, and the range of cultural beliefs and folklore, that always underlie attitudes to illness. Most importantly, that quiet personal story of the patient still needs to be told – and to be listened to with care and compassion. That unique, irreplaceable story of personal illness or suffering, told by a patient to his doctor, and which sometimes emerges slowly or indirectly, often in painful whispers, over very many years. It is those tiny moments of therapeutic intimacy that are at the very core of medical practice. They are what make it such a unique and rewarding profession. But there is a real danger now that among the rush and bustle of techno-medicine, and the buzz of its wonder machines – and all the pressures of bureaucracy, the market, the accountants, and the litigation lawyers – that much of this will eventually be lost.

For all that, this book is in no way a rejection of medical science, nor of its long tradition of experimental enquiry, and the technology that it has produced. For I have always believed that the scientific method is absolutely necessary for any improvement in medical care, and I haven't changed my mind on that.

However, as that great 19th-century physician Sir William Osler made clear, for successful health care Science is absolutely necessary.

But it is also never sufficient.

Cecil Helman

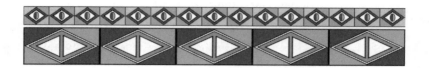

CHAPTER
1

AN AMAZING MURMUR OF
THE HEART

It is 1965, the first year of my clinical studies at the University of Cape Town Medical School, and our very first chance to examine real, live patients in the wards – not just silent cadavers in the dissecting room, or microscope slides in the laboratory. Today, clumps of white-coated medical students are roaming the wards of Groote Schuur Hospital like eager hunter-gatherers. Our prey are what we refer to as 'interesting cases', especially those who are very ill and the bearers of interesting stories, and even more interesting 'physical signs'. It's the only way we can hone our clinical skills, learn how to 'take a history' from a patient, and then examine them, in order to decipher the message hidden behind all those bodily clues. It's the best way to build up our experience of actual disease. At the entrance to one of the male medical wards, a group of us ask one of the junior doctors on duty about whom we should examine. Does he have any 'interesting cases' for us to see? He is busy writing up the patients' charts and occasionally talking on the phone, but he tries to be helpful.

'There's a really interesting spleen,' he says, pointing over his shoulder. 'Third bed on the left. Go and examine it. And then there's that rather interesting pair of lungs in the bed next door. And – best of all – while you're down there, do have a listen to that amazing heart murmur just across the ward from him. Really amazing. It's a mitral stenosis, straight out of a textbook. Have a look at them all. That should keep you busy.'

We thank him and walk through the ward between the long rows of beds, each with a pale, middle-aged man lying in it – some quiet or dozing, others shifting restlessly with pain or apprehension. Many are attached to intravenous drips or monitor machines, while some are surrounded by small clumps of worried relatives. Eventually we find ourselves standing at the foot of the third bed on the left. But instead of a big, black, glistening spleen lying across the bed, there is a small anxious man – a small bald man with 'splenomegaly' (an enlarged spleen), and a complicated tale of increasing weakness, loss of weight, and hard swollen glands in his neck and elsewhere. But we're much less interested in his story, than in his dramatic 'physical sign'. It's his spleen, with its hard, palpable, irregular edge that we're really after.

In the bed next door to him, the pair of lungs looks up at us with a pale, frightened, wheezing face. Of course, there's no pair of moist, pinkish-grey organs to be seen. From behind half-rimmed glasses and a copy of the *Cape Argus*, the owner of the lungs watches us approach his bed. I notice his bluish lips, his tobacco-stained moustache, his heaving, tortured way of breathing, and the way that his fingers are all swollen at their tips, like tiny clubs, each one stained a khaki colour. But what we're really fascinated by are those moist crackling sounds and unusual wheezes from both his lungs, and – when we tap his chest firmly with our fingertips – that irregular area of dullness in the left one. There's something dense and jagged hiding in there, just biding its time.

And then, a while later, on the other side of the ward, there's that 'amazing murmur' – the mitral stenosis, who lies coughing up pink frothy phlegm into a stained handkerchief. He's in his mid-forties, and his face and body are swollen with oedema. A framed picture of two little children stands on the bedside table, smiling at him from a beach somewhere, but he's too ill to smile back at them. There's a tiny vase of flowers, a bottle of guava juice, a Bible, and a neat pile of paperback books besides him. A small bespectacled woman in a floral dress sits quietly at the bedside, reading a religious tract. No matter how hard one looks, there's no scarred, narrowed heart valve in sight. Gasping and coughing, his voicing dropping occasionally to a murmuring sigh, the man tells us that he'd had rheumatic fever as a child, which left him with a damaged mitral valve in his heart. For some time now he's been getting so short of breath that he can't carry on working, and that's why he's recently lost his job. Because he's not earning anything, they've had to dip into their meagre savings, which are almost all gone now. And because he's spending so much time at home these days, that is causing strain between him and his wife (here the woman looks up uneasily), but at this point we've all stopped listening to him. Abruptly he falls silent as, one by one, ignoring what he's saying, we place our stethoscopes firmly onto his clammy chest. It's just as the ward doctor promised – a classic heart murmur. Not the *lub-dub lub-dub* of ordinary heart sounds, but a soft click, and then a *whoosh* of blood, squeezing its way through a narrowed valve, the sound emerging clearly through the earpieces of our stethoscopes. Just as the textbook said it would.

'Hey, so how did it go?' asks the same junior doctor, as we finally leave the ward. 'Man, didn't I tell you what great physical signs they were!'

Yes, it's been a good day, and we are grateful to him. A spleen, a mitral valve murmur, *and* a pair of lungs with a large tumour inside one of them. An embarrassment of riches!

The following year, dressed in loose green trousers, smock and shoe-coverings, I am standing in an operating theatre in the hospital, observing an operation for the first time. The room is tiled in a pastoral green, and the surgeons, anaesthetist and nurses are all wearing the same green-coloured smocks, hats and masks. The air within the room feels cool and disinfected. Except for the low murmur of voices, the clink of instruments, the slow beep-beep-beep of the monitor machines, and the rhythmic puffing of the respirator, nothing else can be heard.

Everyone in the room bar the anaesthetist, busy with his tubes and respirators, is staring at something at the very centre of all this crisp, green foliage. They are concentrating on a pale rectangle, surrounded on each side by green drapes, each one held in place by a shiny silver clip. The rectangle is brightly lit by large circular light suspended from the ceiling, and is being carefully swabbed with a brownish liquid by one of the nurses. Everyone is staring at it. Silently, intently.

Suddenly I notice a faint, slow movement. Up and down, up and down. The rectangle is moving! *The rectangle is breathing*! And furthermore, as the surgeon cuts deeply into it, the rectangle is beginning to bleed. For just a moment I had completely forgotten that this pale, symmetrical area is not just an interesting geometric shape, nor just a rectangular doorway into the hidden secrets of a body. It is actually a part of a person, even though the rest of that person's body is completely hidden from view, especially its head and its face. He is anonymous, unknown, almost irrelevant. All that I know of him is this pale rectangle with the wide gash across its the middle, like a bleeding smile. 'What a tricky gall bladder,' says the surgeon suddenly, his voice echoing off the tiled walls, 'What a real bugger! These bloody gall bladders! Just look at it, all packed with stones and full of pus!'

Another couple of years later, after my graduation, and I am now a young hospital doctor, dutifully following the Consultant on his daily ward round. As he passes in a regal procession from bed to bed, patient to patient, he is trailing behind him – like the ends of an imperial cloak – a long line of white-coated junior doctors, nurses and medical students. Now the focus is not so much on 'physical signs' and surgical rectangles, but more on what I have come to call 'paper patients'. These are the products of diagnostic technology: printouts of blood test results, strips of electrocardiogram paper, X-rays and scans, all filed in the patient's medical folder. At the ward round, these objects, held lovingly in the Consultant's hands, are the real focus of our attention – not poor, terrified Mr R lying in the bed besides us. Frowning, straining to hear what the Consultant is saying about him, he is largely ignored as, standing around the bed, the senior doctors discuss in detail the shadow in his lung, the inverted T-wave in his electrocardiogram, and the low haemoglobin level in his blood tests.

Watching this scene, a question is forming itself in my mind. It's the same, insistent question that's been hovering there for years now, ever since I first began medical school. And it's still there two decades later, but shouted even louder now, one morning in the 1980s when I'm a Visiting Fellow at a famous American medical school. For the first time I am attending one of the weekly Grand Rounds, or clinical case presentations, held at one of its main teaching hospitals. It's a regular opportunity for the senior medical staff to show their most interesting, and puzzling, cases to the rest of us.

By now, the answer to that question – *But where has the patient gone?* – is perfectly obvious. For the human patient has now completely disappeared, atrophied away like a damaged and useless limb, and been replaced only by cells and diseased organs, and by all those slides of 'paper patients' projected onto the screen before us. All that remains of that particular person, that unique case of human suffering, are those rectangular abstractions, the fragments or shards of a shattered human life. Nothing more.

We spend an hour in the big lecture theatre, crowded with white coats and name-tags, listening to one of the Attending Physicians as he carefully presents these fragments to us, one by one, like exhibits in an archaeology museum – a long succession of photographs, slides, scans, X-rays, videotapes and blood tests projected onto the enormous screen behind him. They are like a set of Tarot cards, shuffled on the screen before us, and we watch as the physician cleverly pieces them together into a single message, a coherent whole – decoding the true diagnosis, and likely prognosis, hidden somewhere among them. But despite glancing regularly around the room, I can see no trace of the patient himself. He never appears. All that we have of him is this collage of signs – a semiotic system of his symptoms and physical findings.

Then, at the end of the Grand Rounds, we all get up and leave. The lecture hall empties swiftly. Nothing remains behind us except a few sparse, fading echoes of a particular human life, still projected onto the silent screen.

The young woman lies at the centre of a circle of white coats, and I can sense how the atmosphere around her has begun to thicken. The birthing room has suddenly become tense, stuffy, almost airless. Voices have dropped, the nurses have begun to hurry to and fro, intense, distracted. There is almost no sound except for her gasping breath and occasional moan, the whispered words of her husband, holding her hand, and the rhythmic beep and buzz of the monitor machine. But when I listen more carefully, I can also catch the faint melodic sounds of a Mozart concerto, though at first I'm not sure where it's coming from. Then I realise that she has brought along a small tape-recorder to play at this time, to calm her down during her labour, to help create a more gentle atmosphere. Now it lies thrown on its side, discarded like a useless toy on the small table nearby, hidden behind the large, white, glistening machine that dominates her bedside.

The young couple had hoped for something very different from this, her first birth, and you can see the shock and confusion on their faces. For many months they had attended ante-natal classes in 'natural childbirth' methods – yoga breathing, relaxation exercises, the inner visualisation of peaceful scenes – and yet things have not worked out according to plan. Despite all their preparations, and Mozart, something has gone terribly wrong. She is in the final stages of labour, but that labour is not progressing as it should. It's been going on for many hours now, and still the baby hasn't appeared. Gradually the contractions of her uterus have become sluggish, irregular, weaker by the moment. Her mother, who had hoped to attend the birth, has been sent out of the room, a handkerchief pressed to her face. Everything has suddenly changed.

The young woman's face is flushed and sweating, her green eyes blurry with fatigue. Strands of damp blonde hair cling to her forehead. Her eyes swivel, as if at a tennis match, from us to the pale, taut face of her husband, and then back again. She lies tethered like Gulliver to the bed by a collection of different wires and tubes. She can hardly sit up, or move her body around. As well as the intravenous drip inserted in her wrist, her blood pressure and pulse rate are being monitored continuously by a cuff attached to her other arm. She has also been connected up to the CTG (cardiotocography) machine, and a special sensor leading from it has been strapped to her huge swollen belly, in order to monitor within it the contractions of her ailing uterus, and the heartbeats of her distressed foetus. Lower down, another wire is emerging from within her, linked to a tiny electrode attached to the baby's scalp, still marooned within its exhausted womb.

'Well, there's quite obviously fetal distress,' says the chief obstetrician to our white-coated group, standing on the other side of her bed. 'She's just passed some meconium, and you all know what *that* they means, don't you? Here, let me show you the tracings on the CTG.' I notice that except for a slight nod towards her he is talking to us over her body, bypassing both her and her husband, not making any eye contact with them. He moves around the bed towards that big white machine, with its rows of silver dials, its fluorescent screen and long electric coils.

Like all the others, I am full of admiration for this wondrous object, with its gleaming surfaces and glowing screens, pulsing and buzzing at her bedside. At a critical time like this it is a good ally to have. It's a clever diagnostician, a reliable adviser, an oracle, spewing forth Truth out of its thin, horizontal mouth. It is so helpful to us that all our attention is focused upon it, and what it has to say, as the long white paper printout emerges slowly from within it, the squiggly parallel lines on it recording the baby's heart rate, and the frequency and nature of the uterine contractions. We gather around it, peering closely at the printout, holding it carefully by its edges, closely examining it, commenting to one another on the frequency or irregularity of this squiggle or of that. Someone remarks how the tracing shows that the fetal heart rate is often irregular, how sometimes it beats too fast – well over 170 beats a minute – but occasionally drops to well below 100. The obstetrician reels off facts and figures, a series of numbers and numerical standards, normal and abnormal.

'Basically, it all means the baby is not getting enough oxygen,' he says to us, 'and if we don't operate soon – well, you all *know* what will happen.'

And yet I notice that in all this drama no-one is paying much attention to the woman herself, neither the obstetrician nor ourselves. No-one is asking her or her husband how they are feeling at this moment, or what they make of the situation. No-one seems to be explaining to them exactly what is happening to her body, and to her baby, or what will happen next. Nobody is comforting them, or reassuring them in any way. In fact, for the most part they are ignored by all the focused, frowning medical staff clustered around the bed. The couple seem to have become largely irrelevant. It's as if the woman's body has become merely a soft, unreliable appendage to the hard, but much more reliable machine before us – an appendage that can only be understood by its metallic sister, and not by anyone else.

As each minute passes, and the tension rises, it seems more and more as if this big machine, and not the woman herself, is the true patient today. The focus of all our conversation, the one most entitled to our loving care and attention. It seems to be the one giving birth today, not to a small, wrinkled, crying infant – but to a long strip of white paper, covered with irregular lines.

And yet the obstetrician is not a bad man. I am quite sure of that. He is a kindly person, probably a fine father and a good husband, and an excellent doctor, too. He will do everything he can to deliver the baby safely, and he will probably succeed. But somehow – like so many of my medical tutors before him – the focus of his attention is wrong. He has led us all in the wrong direction, allowing the woman to disappear completely behind the machine, to be obscured by numbers and printouts and statistics. To become almost invisible to our medical gaze.

The spleen, the rectangle, the pair of lungs, that damaged mitral valve. The reams of 'paper patients' handed from doctor to doctor at the bedside, or projected onto a screen in the lecture hall. The data flashing brightly on a computer screen. The tangled web of a genetic code. The young woman in labour, competing for attention with the monitoring machine. In each of these scenes, what remains of the patient is something less than a human being. For, reduced to a meta-language of numbers, symbols and statistics, the ill body seems to have become almost a form of modern art, abstract and stylised. Medical science has become a way of fictionalising the human condition, of reducing it to a much smaller story, and in the process making it seem more distant, less threatening, less disturbing.

I try to think back to the precise point in my medical training when it all began – this process of abstraction and fragmentation. My mind is drawn back, a long time before that Amazing Murmur lying in the ward, to that icy dissecting room, where we were first taught to dismantle the human form – to break it down with our scalpels into its organs, blood vessels, muscles and bones, to turn it into the pieces of a person, with each piece being handled and studied on its own. And yet ironically, as clinical students a year or so later, when we finally came to examine *real* living patients in the hospital wards, we were somehow expected to put all those shattered pieces of Humpty-Dumpty together again – to move rapidly from the part to the whole, from the dead to the living, to reassemble those small fragments into a bigger picture – into something our lecturers increasingly referred to as 'a patient' or 'a person', and not just a collage of bodily parts. It's a difficult task, and some of my classmates would never succeed in doing it. For the rest of their professional lives they would remain focused on only small pieces of people: on the spleen-third-bed-on-the-left, or an even tinier fragments than that.

In that year of our anatomy studies – as we leaned over the icy cadavers, cutting and probing – the pages of our textbooks were filled with graphic illustrations of parts of human bodies, printed in garish colours. These days, thanks to the electron microscope and other developments, those parts are getting even smaller every year. Once filled only with photographs or drawings of organs, blood vessels, bones, muscles, ligaments and nerves, today's anatomy textbooks now also include many more detailed illustrations of its hidden, microscopic structure. Page after page of brightly coloured photographs of various types of cells and their inner components: their nuclei and organelles, and the intricacies of their genetic structure.

Despite this, the main focus in all anatomy books today still remains the individual *organ* – the organ lying on the page, alone, disembodied, in full colour, or in black-and-white, somehow separated from the body in which it normally lives. It's not a new thing. In the original 1858 edition of *Gray's Anatomy* (*'Anatomy: Descriptive and Surgical'*) the vulva, for example, appears in a careful engraving by HV Carver (an appropriate name for an anatomist), as a sort of disembodied life-form. With the Latin words *Labia Majora* and *Labia Minora* superimposed upon it, it is portrayed as a strangely grey oval shape, resembling some complex underwater plant, a type of sea anemone, with its curled pubic fronds swaying in the passing currents. For almost a hundred years that same carefully engraved and disembodied vulva floated through the pages. It was still there in the 27th edition in 1938, though in recent editions it has completely disappeared.

In the same period, the way that these lonely organs are described in the text also seems to have changed, becoming more technical, less lyrical. The 'female organ of copulation' of the 1909 edition has become the 'fibromuscular tube lined with non-keratinized stratified epithelium' of today. The heart, in the 1858 *Gray's Anatomy*, is described as 'a hollow muscular organ, of a conical form, placed between the lungs, and enclosed in the cavity of the pericardium'. By the 39th edition in 2005, with its pages of bright coloured photographs, electron micrographs and CT scans, the description has become crisp and mechanical. Both the 'Placer' and 'Encloser' of the heart have disappeared. 'The heart,' it says simply, 'is a pair of valved muscular pumps combined in a single organ.'

A tube. A pump. A collection of cells. I think that's where it all began.

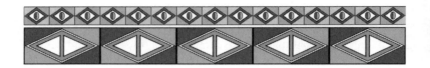

CHAPTER 2

THE MAGIC MACHINE

In 1983, faced with the increasing role of technology in medicine, and its effects on patients, an editorial in the prestigious *Journal of the American Medical Association* posed the question: 'Has the machine become the physician?' 'The fact that the health care provided in the system may be improved as a result of the technology,' wrote *JAMA*, 'does not have as much impact as the subtle and hidden message that the machine has become the physician: the definitive adviser. The specialist-physician is metamorphosing into a technocrat and a businessman. The physician retreats behind the machine, and becomes an extension of the machine.'

Young Dr A, keen and intelligent, is an example of this new breed of doctor – the ones I call 'techno-doctors'. He is an avid computer fan, as well as a physician. He likes nothing better than to sit in front of his computer screen, hour after hour, peering at it through his horn-rimmed spectacles, tap-tapping away at its keyboard. It's a magic machine, for it contains within itself its own small, finite, rectangular world, a brightly coloured abstract landscape of signs and symbols. It seems to be a world that is much easier for Dr A to understand, and much easier for him to control, than the real world – one largely without ambiguity or emotion. It is in this micro-world that he chooses to deal with a very different type of patient – one that is actually not there, someone who has no corporeal existence at all, and who exists mostly as a set of electronic signals in cyberspace. Certainly not someone whom he ever needs to touch or embrace, or to feel that someone's warm skin or pulse, or to listen carefully to its story of suffering.

Like many other doctors of his generation – though fortunately still only a minority – Dr A prefers to see people and their diseases mainly as digital data, which can be stored, analysed, and then, if necessary, transmitted – whether by internet, telephone or radio – from one computer to another. He is one of those helping to create a new type of patient, and a new type of patient's body – one much less human and tangible than those cared for by his medical predecessors. It is one stage further than reducing the body down to a damaged heart valve, an enlarged spleen or a diseased pair of lungs. For this 'post-human' body is one that exists mainly in an abstract, immaterial form. It is a body that has become pure *information*.

Thanks to medical technology, from the humble stethoscope up to the sophisticated MRI scans of today, physicians like Dr A can now by-pass the patient almost completely. They can go straight to the body, measuring and analysing its inner workings, without even having to listen to the patients themselves. With the aid of this equipment, they can now pinpoint, with far greater accuracy than ever before, the exact location and nature of the pathology, and then decide how to treat it. And where doctors from previous generations once listened attentively to the stories their patients told them about their physical state, as well as their personal lives, their fears and hopes, as far as Dr A is concerned, all of this is meaningless noise. It's as if he is perpetually tuned into the wrong wave-length. Where the others could once hear human speech, and the messages that it conveyed, all he can hear is static – random, meaningless, irritating sound. It is without meaning to him. It is not language at all.

A friend of mine, born with a hereditary condition known as polycystic kidney disease (PKD) tells me of his visits to the renal clinic at his local hospital, and his own encounter with a version of Dr A. The disease only manifested itself in my friend's body in his mid-40s, but now, several years later, his kidneys have begun to fail, their normal structure gradually replaced by an archipelago of small cysts growing within them. They are increasingly unable to clear his blood of its waste products, to keep its levels of salts and chemicals at their normal levels, and to produce an adequate supply of urine. He has developed severe chronic renal failure, and his blood pressure is rising precipitously. Now dialysis waits in the wings and possibly, one day, a kidney transplant as well. He realises that if he has to undergo the dialysis, everything about his lifestyle will have to change – his work pattern too. For at least three times a week, and for three to four hours at a time, he will be forced to join his body to an alien machine, to become one half of a cyborg – a reluctant Siamese twin.

But the kidneys are not the only thing failing in his life. Several months before this time, his young wife died tragically of a rare form of cancer, and he is now the sole supporter of their young child. He needs a life. He needs to work, to earn money, to mix with other people, and to be there to support his child emotionally, as well as financially. The wounds of his wife's death are still raw. At least for a while, he needs to experience the semblance of a normal life. But as his kidneys slowly fail, he is becoming even more anxious each time he visits the clinic, his mind increasingly full of questions and worries. And yet the bespectacled young doctor behind the desk seems to be completely uninterested in all of this. Each time he sees my friend at the clinic, they go through the same, almost identical, ritual. There is a brief greeting, a brief examination, some blood is taken from his arm, and then immediately all the attention in the room switches to the computer on the doctor's desk. For that luminescent rectangle is the real focus of the consultation. It is the real doctor, as well as the real patient – and a more manageable one at that. First tap-tapping away at the keyboard, the doctor brings up on the screen the results of my friend's most recent blood tests. Each time, staring at the screen, the young man in the white coat reels off from it a list of figures: the latest levels of the creatinine, urea, electrolytes, sugar and haemoglobin in his bloodstream, as well as his blood pressure and other measures – a lengthy list of numbers. Amidst all of this numerology, this fog of statistics and probabilities that he is being given, my friend tries to raise some of his other concerns. About his personal life, his son, his job, his many worries for the future, and how he feels about it all. But each time he speaks the doctor looks at him blankly through his thick lenses, mumbles a few words, and then with relief turns swiftly back to the computer screen, tap-tapping away. My friend has the feeling that, for this doctor at least, he is not really present in the room. He has become merely a translucent spectre, only partially visible. He has been reduced not only to a pair of ailing kidneys, but also to a series of numbers – a long series of fluorescent numbers leaping off the computer screen, and then flowing swiftly to and fro across the desk. From the machine into the doctor's mind – and then back again.

For all its reduction by medical technology, the human body as por-trayed in *Gray's Anatomy*, and other anatomy textbooks, has always been a solid thing – a firm, material object. Something you could touch and handle. Something with weight and texture and smell. Something you could see lying in the ward, or being dissected in the anatomy lab. For centuries, this solid object has been at the very core of medical science. But even that has recently begun to change, and the techno-doctors are partly to blame.

Today many medical schools, especially in North America, have become fans of the 'Visible Human Project' (VHP), begun in 1989 by the United States National Library of Medicine. It consists of an online library of thousands of digital images, many of them three-dimensional, based mainly on multiple MRI and CT scans of the bodies of two dead people: an adult male and an adult female. These detailed anatomical images (or 'computerized cadavers', as someone has called them) are now available to licensees in 48 countries, where they are used for educational, diagnostic and research purposes. More and more medical students and doctors are now learning about the inner structure of the human body, not from examining living patients, nor from dissecting dead ones, but from the computer screen.

They can also learn about the body's genetic structure from the 'Human Genome Project' (HGP), completed in 2003 at a cost of about three billion US dollars. It is a vast mapping of all the DNA contained in the human organism, and the results are also available online. Bioethicists have begun to warn against the growing use of the computer imagery in genetics, especially the way that the individual's genetic inheritance (their 'genetic code') is being increasingly described as if it were some sort of software program – one which helps build the body, makes it function, and which, under certain circumstances, may be modifiable by 'genetic engineering'. Genes themselves are described as if they were tiny storage units, much like computer micro-chips, containing large amounts of information about that individual's past, present and likely future. Genetic diseases, like computer viruses, therefore become primarily 'diseases of information' – rather than diseases of people, and their bodies. As the philosopher JJ Rheinberger has put it, the central dogma of this approach can be summarised as: 'DNA makes RNA, RNA makes protein.' In his view, it's a limited, impoverished view of the human organism as primarily 'a medium of communication and control', one whose functions are largely determined by 'genetically enshrined instruction'.

Such genetic determinism is not without cost. It can over-emphasise the role of genes in human behaviour, especially their influence on intelligence, race, gender and unconventional lifestyles, as well as on physical and mental illness. It can lead one to largely ignore the role of more personal and psychological factors in shaping human experience, and the response to illness and suffering. It also represents a shift away from examining changeable social and environmental influences towards an abstract map of less changeable biological mechanisms. It's a change in how we actually conceptualise 'a person', and it can result in the loss of some ancient sense of what it means it be human.

For all their undoubted benefits to medicine, and to medical education, some have criticised the VHP and the HGP, seeing them both as being radical re-conceptualisations of the human body – not as living flesh-and-blood, but mainly as digital data. Writing in the journal *Advances in Nursing Science*, Margarete Sandalowski has noted that: 'The body in these projects is data come to life on our computer screens.' Both projects allow entry into these virtual bodies without actually opening up, and touching, a living human body. And both help create yet another form of 'post-human' body, one which she describes as 'a disembodied informational structure with no clearly defined self'. In her view, the true hidden cost of this process is 'the disappearance of the humanist body, of the flesh-and-blood encasing of a unique and stable self'.

In *The Second Self*, the psychologist Sherry Turkle has come to the same conclusion. She shows how increasing numbers of people – much like Dr A, perhaps – now regard their computer as not just a physical object, but also as an anthropomorphic 'thinking machine', a sort of extra brain outside their body. With our increasing involvement with these devices, there is now a blurring of boundaries between computer and owner, with each subtly influencing the other. For that reason, Turkle poses two questions about this novel situation: 'What happens when people consider the computer as a model of human mind?' she asks, and – perhaps more importantly – 'What happens when people begin to think they are machines?' Seeing the mind as merely a 'software program' (capable thus of being 're-programmed') that is located within the 'hardware' of the skull, can lead to a very different conception of human identity. Like Sandalowski, she sees how this view of the 'mind as microprocessor' can leave one with the sense of 'a decentralized self', a sense that there is actually no 'I', no 'me'; no unitary 'conscious actor' at the very core of one's being – just a collection of actions and processes. Above all, it is the sense of a hollow self, of an emptiness at the very core of mind and body, of being somehow 'run' from the outside like some complex machine.

In fact, compared with the wondrous machines of medicine, the human body is a rather inadequate, rather inferior, soft machine. Its brain is less efficient than a computer, its bones more brittle than those made of titanium; a dialysis machine is more predicable than a human kidney, cardiac pacemakers beat more regularly than an old-fashioned human heart. In order to function better, the human body now needs help. It needs to be enhanced and improved with the aid of medical science and technology. It needs artificial organs, spare parts made of steel, plastic, rubber or nylon. It's become an almost robotic creature, robbed of autonomy and humanity. When it's ill, it needs an engineer, not a doctor.

To many techno-doctors, medicine thus is all about 'synecdoche' – that is, where the part comes to stand for, or represent, the whole. They believe that it's all that they need to know, even though the size of that bodily part they do know is shrinking rapidly. From the spleen-third-bed-on-the-left down to a particular disease process ('that heart failure in bed number two'), it has since shrunk even further to specific organs or cells, even an unruly molecule or two. Furthermore, for some super-specialists, the part now actually *is* the whole. Those small fragments of a patient that they deal with, revealed by their diagnostic machines, have become patients in their own right. A damaged heart, a swollen liver, an enlarged spleen, an inadequate pancreas, a list of numbers on the computer screen, will sometimes receive closer attention from them than any ill person ever could.

But the part is never quite the whole. My friend in the renal clinic, the young woman in the birthing room, that amazing murmur lying in the medical ward, all answer the question I first began asking back in medical school, many years ago: *'But where has the patient gone?'* The answer they give is obvious: they have gone nowhere. They have not disappeared or atrophied away, nor been buried under a mountain of statistical probabilities, nor reduced to a wavy line on a graph, a shadow on an X-ray plate, a slide of cellular structure. They are still here, still staring hopefully up at their doctors from their hospital beds, or from across the medical desk. They are still here, waiting for their doctors to notice them again, to shift their attention away from all their magic machines and their high-tech toys, their fascination with molecules and enzymes and collections of numbers. And to bear witness to their suffering and anxiety, and then to do what they can to relieve them. Above all, to listen to their stories again. And – hidden among those stories – to hear the faint, almost inaudible, murmuring of their hearts.

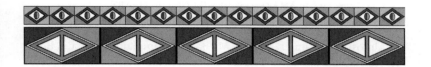

CHAPTER 3

THE *DYBBUK* OF EDDIE BARNETT

At the time that I knew him, Eddie Barnett was the bearer of a strange story, one that wandered continuously from one part of his body to another. But whether that story originated in the depths of his own subconscious, or from somewhere else, I never really found out.

Despite the passing of decades, I can still see him sitting across the desk from me, moaning softly, his hand moving about his body, tightly gripping one part, then soothing another. He is in his late 60s, long divorced, and has several children living abroad with whom he has little contact. He is a lonely man, with the look about him of a man without women – certainly of someone who has not shared his life with a woman for very many years. When he comes to consult me at the Medical Centre, he usually wears a long grey coat, whatever the season, pulled over a darkish jacket, slightly frayed at the cuffs and collar. His mouth is always turned downwards at the corners, like an inverted moon. His haircut is always indifferent, his beard and moustache ragged and irregularly streaked with grey. A deep frown divides his forehead into a grid of vertical and horizontal fissures. Under his jacket, the shirts that he wears are crumpled and un-ironed. On several occasions I notice that some of the buttons have been left undone, or been inserted into the wrong button-holes.

Almost every time I see him, Mr Barnett complains of a pain. But it is a pain unlike any other pain I have ever encountered. He describes it to me in vivid, dynamic terms. 'Well, at the moment, doctor, it's basically in my neck, but it often moves over to my shoulders, especially the right one. Now I can feel it in the curvature of my spine. No, no, a bit lower down than that, more in my lower back, right here near the bottom. Sometimes it moves into my stomach, here, or sometimes here, or in my bladder. But sometimes it begins to pinch on one side of my face, like so, and then moves to the same side of my body.' He always carries with him a full portfolio of adjectives. Some days the pain is 'sharp' and 'intense', on other days 'dull and constant', or merely a 'vague ache' or 'discomfort'. In turn it is 'heavy', 'shooting', 'burning', 'stabbing', 'shocking' or 'throbbing'. Sometimes it is accompanied by other symptoms, such as a headache, vague tummy aches, or feelings of stiffness in his neck, shoulders, or in one leg or the other.

Mr Barnett speaks of his pain all the time. He seems obsessed with it. Consultations with him always leave me feeling frustrated, exhausted, drained of energy. He follows every suggestion I make with another question, and one after that. Asking him for more details of his pain provokes even more requests for help, and then more after that. He is insatiable, unsatisfiable – like an elderly bearded baby, sucking desperately at an emptied breast.

And yet every medical test he's had so far has shown no physical abnormality whatsoever. He has been blood tested, X-rayed, scoped, scanned, monitored and probed by hospitals and pain clinics all over the city. But each time the tests prove negative.

I offer to refer him to a psychiatrist, a therapist, a counsellor, even a priest, but he always refuses.

'There's nothing wrong with me up here,' he says emphatically, tapping his forehead. 'I'm not mad. It's just that I've got this terrible pain that will not go away. Do you understand? It's the *pain* that's giving me depression. Not the other way round.'

Months go by. Pointless, frustrating months. None of my treatments seem to work, none of my pain-killers. And then, as time goes on, I begin to notice something about the unusual way he refers to his pain. It is that he always groups his disparate symptoms into a single, painful entity, and then describes this malign essence as an 'It'. As if it were a foreign Thing, an abstract being with its own volition, its own malevolent personality.

'Now *it* has moved to my other shoulder,' he says, or, 'Now *it's* boring right through my chest.' '*It* won't let me sleep at night,' he says, 'and *it's* making me depressed,' '*It's* driving me mad.' He speaks as if this entity has singled him out. For some unknown reason, it has chosen to enter his body, and to take up residence among his organs and cells, and then to torture him mercilessly for so many years. '*It's* killing me, doctor,' he says, again and again, '*It's* really torturing me.'

More pain-killers, more futile advice. Still no improvement. But despite this apparent lack of success, I gradually become aware that something *is* happening to the pain during our meetings. Something of what I say to him *is* being heard – at least on the bodily level. For I notice that often, in response to one of my suggestions (especially one that is particularly emphatic), the pain suddenly comes to life. It seems for a while to go berserk. It begins to leap frantically around his body, like a caged animal trying to escape. It appears first in one part of his body, then swiftly in another. Burrowing in and out of different areas of his head or chest or abdomen with amazing rapidity – sinking then emerging, chewing its way out of this joint or that limb like a demented beaver.

If Eddie Barnett and I had been living in one of those more traditional, tribal societies – the ones I'd learned about during my anthropology studies, shortly after medical school – I might have called in an exorcist or a shaman to remove his pain, and not a psychotherapist. But instead of a ritual of feathers, drums or holy relics, he has had to make do with a young, inexperienced family doctor. And also with all those white-coated specialists at the hospital to whom he's been referred, and who have also brandished their stethoscopes, syringes and tablets at him – all without effect.

A year goes by, without any change. My treatments are pointless, my medical textbooks quite useless. I begin to delve instead into all those books on my shelf on folklore and anthropology. And to pay much more attention to the characteristics of the pain itself, for when I do so a sort of identikit slowly emerges. A profile of the 'It'. One day I sit down and write out a list of every one of the attributes of its complex, and rather unique 'personality' that have manifested themselves in my office over time. And then I understand why that pain had sometimes seemed so familiar. For as Eddie Barnett described it – and as the pain itself spoke, indirectly, yet audibly through him – it was actually the mirror-image of his own personality. In fact, everything that Eddie Barnett is, the pain *is not*.

Where Eddie is rigid, his body hardly moving beyond its tense, frozen posture – the pain is mobile. It moves here, dances there, flying swiftly from one part of his body to another, quicker than the eye could follow. Where he is uncreative, unable to formulate any new ideas or new ways of living his life – the pain is cunning and intelligent. It is endlessly creative in its invention of new forms, new appearances, new ways of dancing among the limbs and organs of his body. Where he is dull and boring, his voice flat and monotonous – the pain seems to live an exciting life. It clearly has a temperament that is vibrant and versatile, one full of surprises. Where he is almost moribund, in an emotional and social sense – the pain is very much alive. In fact, it seems to be looking forward to an even longer life, within its warm, mobile, comfortable home. Where Eddie is frozen in his unhappiness, unable to make any decisions, or decide what to do – the pain is endlessly innovative. There is no end to its ingenuity, and to the strategies that it has designed to defeat the doctors. Where he is passive, fatalistic and defeated by life and its many vicissitudes – the pain fights back. Its survival instincts are evidently powerful, and never seem to slacken. It is active in self-defence. It intervenes in history. It outwits – again and again – those like myself who would drive it out into the wilderness. And finally, where Eddie is stifled and often inarticulate – the pain is garrulous. Nothing can halt its talkativeness, its endless flow of colourful images in its chosen language – the dialect of symptoms.

Like so many other symptoms in medical practice, that pain is telling a story.

Most doctors would label Eddie Barnett as a classic example of the so-called 'pain-prone patient' – one of those sad, disturbed individuals, often filled with feelings of guilt or self-blame, who suffer not from any physical disease, but from a 'psychogenic pain' produced by their own unconscious mind. People who feel, deep down, that they really deserve to suffer.

But it's a limited view. The picture here is deeper, and more nuanced than that. From an anthropological perspective, the same picture could look very different. For Eddie Barnett could be seen as personifying, or embodying, a very common metaphor for the cause of suffering. It's a universal trope, the feeling of having been 'possessed' or 'entered' by some malevolent, invisible force (the 'It' in his case); an alien entity that somehow enters one and then causes physical or mental illness or other misfortune. It's an idea that is remarkably common in peoples and cultures throughout the world, from tribal groups to modern industrial societies. While we in the West tend to blame invisible 'germs' or 'pollutants' for many of our health problems (though some still see cancer as a malevolent 'invasion' from without), beliefs about 'spirit possession' remain common in some less developed parts of Africa, Asia and Latin America.

In those more traditional settings, blaming 'possession' by evil spirits can be seen as a folk explanation for unexplained illness, for unexpected changes in behaviour, or for more serious conditions such as schizophrenia. But the quirky nature of Eddie Barnett's pain reminds me instead of one type of 'spirit possession' in particular.

It is the legend of the *dybbuk*.

This curious mythological being is a familiar figure in Jewish folklore and cabbalistic thought, from the Middle Ages onwards. More recently, it makes an appearance in the work of Isaac Bashevis Singer, in stories like *The Dead Fiddler* and *Satan in Goray*. It is usually described as the restless, wandering soul of a dead person that somehow enters or 'possesses' a living person against that person's will. Often it is the soul of a sinner, or of one who has died prematurely. Sometimes, as in the play *The Dybbuk* by S Ansky, it is the soul of a jilted lover, possessing his intended bride on the day of her wedding to another man. Some cabbalists saw *dybbuks* as souls who had failed to complete their cycle of reincarnation or transmigration, striving for a higher state with each incarnation – an idea not unlike those of Buddhism and Hinduism. For some reason, instead of reincarnating itself, it now temporarily possesses a body that already has a soul of its own, in order to either uplift or punish it.

Whatever its origin, once it has entered its new body and taken up residence there as a sort of malevolent second-self, the *dybbuk* declares its presence. Like a ventriloquist, it begins to speak and to act through its victim, revealing its identity by the symptoms that it causes – pain, cramps, paralysis and many others. There may also be a sudden change in voice, personality, demeanour or behaviour. In Singer's story *The Dead Fiddler*, for instance, the body of a young girl, frail, shy, withdrawn and neurotic, is entered by Getsl, the *dybbuk* of a long-dead fiddler: a tough, streetwise character and heavy drinker, full of lewd jokes and vile obscenities – a being who is the complete opposite in every way (just like Eddie Barnett's pain) of her former demure personality.

Getting rid of this unpleasant invader usually involves a divinatory séance carried out by a religious figure or traditional healer – someone who first identifies the offending spirit, then exorcises it by prayer and ritual to restore the victim to health.

There is one major difference, though, between the *dybbuk* and most other forms of spirit possession – and that's the reason why it reminds me so closely of Eddie Barnett's unusual pain. For in folklore, most of these other malign spirits are, as it were, generic – mass-produced by the culture from which they arise. They tend to have stereotyped personalities, with each type of spirit causing very similar symptoms in all their victims, speaking through them all in that same, recognisable, demonic voice. Most of them lack the quirky, raucous individuality of the *dybbuk*. Unlike most of the others, the *dybbuks* appear to have a distinct vitality about them. They are dead, but they are also very much alive. They may have gruff voices and harsh tones, cause pain, chaos and consternation, but they almost always have a story to tell – sometimes tragic, at others times comic. Each seems to have its own distinctive personality, its own specific needs and desires. In folktales, male *dybbuks* often like an occasional glass of vodka or *schnapps*, as well as a pretty girl, content to possess her warm female body through the long, wintry East European nights. Unlike those mournful grey spectres – also the restless, wandering souls of the dead – that float through the pages of British ghost stories, they seem more sociable, preferring the intimacy of a living body to wandering alone through cold, dark, empty houses carrying their heads under their arms, or rattling their chains.

Those two types of mythological being – the ghost and the *dybbuk* – can both be seen as images of what psychotherapists would call 'unfinished business'. Both have something incomplete, unfulfilled about them.

Usually they've had their earthly existence cut off suddenly, prematurely, together with all their hopes, fears, dreams and intentions. Circumstances have never allowed them to fully mature, to flower into all their personal potential. Often this has been the result of a sudden, early death – by suicide (especially after a doomed love affair), or by murder, accident or war. Unable ever to grow older or wiser, none of these invisible creatures can ever really 'rest easily'. They will reappear, again and again, until their unfinished business is completed.

For those mournful 're-enactment ghosts' – with their dreamy, distracted air – who seem compelled to repeatedly act out their original suffering, it is often a compulsion, as the folklorist Katherine M Briggs puts it, to 'warn, admonish, punish, or protect the living, to impart important information to them, or to ritually re-enact their own deaths'. They symbolise therefore the voice of conscience, and the punitive powers of memory and guilt. But often they are also the bearers of secrets, the tellers of tales. Many have something to 'get off their chests', even though those chests are transparent as air.

This type of ghost usually continues to haunt the actual site of its tragic death, dressed in the same clothing, and behaving in exactly the same way – as if by doing so, it can eventually erase that original pain. Like second-rate thespians, hired at the lowest fee from some failing theatrical agency, these ghosts seem to have only a limited repertoire – acting out the same scene, over and again, even after the audience has long gone home to bed.

As with the ghost of Hamlet's murdered father, those spectres are:

Doom'd for a certain term to walk the night
And for the day confin'd to fast in fires
Till the foul crimes done in my days of nature
Are burnt and purg'd away.

And just like so many human neurotics, they seem to be trapped in a time-warp of their own unhappy pasts. Firmly stuck in past pains, and unable to grow or to move on, they have a compulsion to replay that original suffering, over and over again. In this, many ghost tales echo Sigmund Freud's remark about the neurotic's 'compulsion to repeat' past traumatic experiences, in order to heal them. 'The repetition,' he wrote, 'can take the form of dreams, storytelling, or even hallucination'. It can also take place by 'acting out' those past traumas. Ghosts, though, can be seen as images not only of unresolved trauma, but of inner conflicts made visible. Unlike the more internalised *dybbuk* of Eddie Barnett, they have a shadowy existence in the world outside the body. They are in a sense *extra-corporeal neuroses*. Thus Macbeth's anguished cry:

'Hence, horrible shadow! Unreal mock'ry, hence!'

could easily be the cry of any psychotherapist, striving to rid her client of the haunting memories, and recurrent echoes, of some early childhood trauma.

And for the several years that I knew Eddie Barnett, it could have been my cry as well.

In purely medical terms, Eddie Barnett is a therapeutic disaster. Every attempt to free him from his pain has ended in failure. As a doctor, I cannot exorcise him, 'lay the ghost', shock him with electrical currents, or expel the pain out of his little toe like some traditional healers used to do. And the origin of his *dybbuk* remains a perpetual mystery to me, the nature of that 'unfinished business' still obscure. Was his personal *dybbuk*, I often wonder, perhaps the embodiment of his angry ex-wife, or of someone else from his distant past, still haunting him from within? Early on I find that there's no point in interrogating him directly about this, for he always remains coy and elusive, choosing only to reply in a cryptic language of moans and grimaces, of muscular twitches and clutched abdomens.

So over time, and rather reluctantly, I learn to abandon my medical textbook view of him, and to escape from the cul-de-sac of 'psychogenic pain'. In any case, I have come to see his eccentric pain as much more interesting than that. I return instead to my more anthropological, folkloric view of him. And in doing so I recall, as well, the comments of the psychoanalyst Joyce McDougall about her own pain-prone patients. How for some of them, physical illness, however unpleasant, may be experienced as reassuring proof that, on some level, they are still capable of feeling, that they still exist. 'A body that suffers,' she writes, 'is also a body that is alive.'

Gradually that medical model of symptom and treatment, disease and cure – the one I'd always been trained to apply – falls away. I stop trying to rid him of his pain. For those failures of treatment all seem to be saying the same thing, telling me the same story. It's the real message of his pain. 'Let me be', it seems to be saying, 'just let me live'.

And so, very slowly, Eddie and I develop a new sort of *modus vivendi*, a tacit agreement between us that I will abandon all attempts to destroy or expel his pain, while he will go through the regular ritual of trying one pain-killer after another, and of occasionally 'making progress' for my benefit – at least for a while. Our meetings take on the character of a double consultation: one with Eddie Barnett, and the other with his Pain. There is reassurance and explanation for Eddie, some chemical food for the Pain.

Months go by. Eventually a sort of sad calm begins to descend on him. He seems to gradually make a melancholy peace with his invisible *doppelganger*, his vibrant and versatile twin, the painful *dybbuk* that he has created within himself. The civil war raging inside himself seems to calm. At times he seems even cheerful. He even smiles a little. I realise that all along I have been quite wrong about him, and about his social situation. He is not, after all, as lonely as he first seemed, a man without a woman. For unlike so many other people who have passed through my office, he is never entirely alone. However unpleasant the relationship with the Pain may be, he has a constant and intimate companion. Someone who shares his body, as well as his bed. Eddie Barnett is certainly not as isolated as he appeared to be.

Now our consultations become increasingly a form of marital therapy – teaching him how to live with his personal *dybbuk* in relative harmony. And encouraging him slowly to develop, with the aid of this drug or that, a certain way of living contentedly with the dynamic, yet painful, other half of himself.

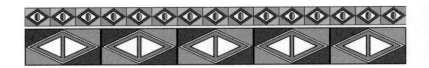

CHAPTER
4

STORIES LIKE THE WIND

In my native South Africa, the San people – once known as the Bushmen, and the original inhabitants of the land – have a rich oral tradition, one that has lasted for millennia. For all that time, their traditional stories and myths have been told, and re-told, around their crackling campfires, the sparks rising up to join the huge canopy of stars in the dense African night. These stories were usually about great hunts or great heroes, but also about mythical animals and man-animals. Stories told while in the deep shadows of the veldt around them, they could hear the rustle and roar of unseen creatures.

For the San, stories had an existence separate from that of their teller. They were believed to inhabit the physical landscape around them. They were everywhere. Stories floated around on the wind. They passed through mountains and travelled across the veldt, carrying the story from one story-teller to the next. The stories drifted especially to those who were alert to them, and could take them in – and then tell them to the rest of the tribe, before they moved on to the next teller. As one San elder back in the 1870s put it, 'I listen, watching for a story, which I want to hear… I sit waiting for it; that it may float into my ear.' 'I feel a story is the wind', he said.

Each re-telling of a mythic story was unique, a performance tailored to a particular audience, at a particular time and place. The story told was always the same, but at the same time it was always very different.

The story that the wind blows into my office that Monday morning seems at first to be a familiar one. Only later does it turn into something very different.

Sitting across the desk from me is a bald and broad-shouldered man with a worried face. Gary is in his middle 40s, a married man with three children. He works 'somewhere in advertising'. I am much younger than him, and completely new to family practice.

Speaking quickly and breathlessly, and sighing frequently, he says that he is very worried. In the previous few days he has had several episodes of severe pain on the left side of his chest, each one lasting about five minutes. He is worried that it 'may have something to do with my heart'. He says he's been under a lot of stress recently, with problems at work, financial worries, the illness of his elderly mother, the long drive to work, and the lack of sleep caused by a new baby.

I write all this down, and then examine him fully, but I find nothing wrong. But have I missed something? It's the same question that hovers in my mind every day, ever since I first began in clinical practice. Have I overlooked the subtle warning signs of something serious? Perhaps of an imminent heart attack? My anxiety leads me to refer him urgently to a cardiologist at the local hospital, for a specialist opinion.

'I'm sure there's nothing seriously wrong with you,' I say to him, as I hand him the referral letter. 'I'm sure the pain you've had was just due to muscle strain, but ... anyway, we'd better make quite sure and have a few tests done today at the hospital.'

Later I learn from his wife Michelle what happened next. In the Emergency Department of the hospital he's examined by a young intern, even younger and more inexperienced than I am, who does an electrocardiogram and takes some blood tests. Again nothing abnormal is found, but the young doctor is also anxious. He, too, seems to be worried that he may be missing something; something subtle, half-hidden. A short time later, to Gary's dismay, he is admitted to the Intensive Care Unit. Here he finds himself, now trembling with anxiety, lying among rows of silent, elderly men with pale-grey clammy faces and laboured breathing, each one linked to an intravenous drip and wired up to monitor machines. Soon he too is wired up, tethered tightly to machines on all sides, and a cannula is inserted in his arm. For three days he is kept like that in a bed in the Unit, and hardly permitted to move. He is constantly examined by a bustling succession of doctors, nurses and technicians, and many more tests are done on him. The doctors who come to his bedside during this time all ask him the same set of questions, again and again: 'Is the pain like a pressure in your chest?' they ask. 'Does it feel like a tight iron band?' 'Does it travel to your left shoulder, then down your left arm?' 'Does it travel up to your neck, or through to your back?' 'Are you short of breath?' 'Do you feel cold and sweaty?'

One of the busy junior doctors tells him, while rushing past his bed, that he's 'probably had a mild heart attack'. And then writes me a quick note stating that Gary had suffered a 'myocardial infarction'. I read the letter with sympathy, then file it away.

Later, Gary is transferred for ten days to a larger ward where everyone else is also a 'heart case'. For the first three days here he is forbidden to walk, and can only go to the toilet in a wheelchair, accompanied by a nurse.

Then something miraculous happens. To his amazed relief, he is told by a more senior doctor in the ward that the initial diagnosis was actually incorrect. The tests show that he has *not*, in fact, had a heart attack. It seems the junior doctor who saw him at first jumped too quickly to the wrong conclusions – one that became a sort of self-fulfilling prophecy. But he has reviewed the case carefully, and come to a different conclusion. But just as Gary is leaving the room, feeling light and airy with relief inside, he hears the doctor add, almost as an afterthought, 'But you probably have angina.'

He is silent as his wife drives him home, completely deflated now, like a balloon pricked by an unexpected needle. He carries home with him a large supply of nifedipine, a drug commonly used to treat angina,

He has been told not to work for at least six weeks.

A week or two later, and Michelle comes to see me at the office. Holding a handkerchief tightly crumpled in one hand, she says she's become increasingly worried about Gary. Ever since he's returned home, he's been feeling unwell. He's over-anxious and physically exhausted. He is shuffling slowly around the house, alert to the slightest changes in his body, with one hand held carefully to his chest, freezing in panic at the slightest discomfort anywhere in that region. His condition seems to be deteriorating every day, she says. For in these last few days, he's started to develop episodes of left-sided chest pain again, increasingly severe each time, and which can last up to seven or eight hours at a time. He describes the pain to her as being like a 'pressure', much like a tight iron band constricting his chest. It travels often to his neck, to his left shoulder, and then down his left arm, and sometimes into his jaw or even through to his back. He is easily tired, often short of breath. Often, he says, his skin feels cold and sweaty. He has become increasingly nervous about doing anything physical, and just stays at home most days, watching television. Shaking her head, she tells that he's becoming apathetic, withdrawn, terrified that he will never lead a normal life again, that soon he will die.

To clear up this diagnostic riddle (the hospital letter that accompanied him home also said Gary's pain 'was thought to be anginal in origin'), he is sent to a private cardiologist for further tests. This eminent doctor, a tall man with half-moon glasses and a large practice in the centre of town, examines him thoroughly, and does numerous tests on him, including several electrocardiograms and an angiogram. And then, smiling gently, he reassures Gary and his wife that he does *not* have any heart disease. None at all. The tests he's done are 95 per cent reliable, he says, and they all show *no* evidence of a heart attack, and none of angina. The hospital doctors, with their 'probably' and 'thought to be', and their loose talk about his being a 'heart case', had worried him unduly. Perhaps due to their inexperience, and their fears of missing a diagnosis and of then being sued, they had opted too much on the side of caution. They had given him a physical diagnosis, but without any physical evidence to support it.

Instead, the eminent cardiologist says that, clearly, Gary has what he terms '*pseudo-angina*'. He explains that it's a type of muscular-skeletal chest pain, probably brought on by stress and anxiety, and made worse by hyper-ventilation – the rapid, panting breaths of an anxiety attack. It can closely mimic heart disease but, fortunately, it's not the real thing. He reassures them that 'there is no evidence of ischaemic heart disease whatsoever.'

When he hears this, Michelle tells me that Gary immediately looks '20 years younger'. For a while his symptoms disappear almost completely. He is still worried about this or that, but he says to her, gratefully, that the cardiologist has finally put his mind at rest.

But the story doesn't end there. For Gary doesn't quite return fully to a normal life. At least, not yet. For a long time afterwards he remains anxious and pale. The stress in his personal life is still there, and despite the doctor's reassurance he occasionally still suspects 'that something is radically wrong with my body'. Sometimes he has vague chest pain again. Sometimes he feels weak. Sometimes he feels tense about 'not breathing properly'. He has become nervous again about over-exerting himself, and about travelling long distances from home. Tightly clutching another handkerchief, Michelle describes how, ever since his time in the Intensive Care Unit, he's become a changed person.

'He's still not himself,' she says, shaking her head. 'He's turned into someone else'.

Gary has acquired a new disease; one I call a *pseudo-disease*. It's a new story that he's heard about himself, and about the vulnerability, and possible defects, of his own body. It's the type of story that these days drifts increasingly between the worlds of doctors and those of patients, and then back again. It's about angina and heart attacks, and the 'typical' types of symptoms that one would expect to accompany them.

It's a story that exists quite separately from the story-teller, and has often existed long before they were born, and will continue long after they have gone. It usually begins its long journey in medical textbooks, but then gradually migrates outwards into the community. It becomes a type of social contagion carried on the wind. It can circulate through a family, a neighbourhood or a city, or even an entire country. Sometimes it can take the form of an epidemic of mass hysteria sweeping through a group of young schoolgirls, collapsing one after another with identical symptoms of vomiting, pains, palpitations or weakness. A pseudo-disease can even begin in one part of the world, and then move on to another, spread like a virulent virus by television or radio, or by the internet – which can produce its own type of hypochondria, known as 'cyberchondria'. It can spread by magazines and newspapers, and by countless conversations in the park or the pub. Some learn about it from other people. Some learn it directly from their doctors.

Pseudo-diseases can be just as contagious as viruses, sometimes even more so. I know that from experience. At medical school many of us suffered from recurrent bouts of a different type of contagion known as 'Medical Students Disease'. It's a common form of hypochondria afflicting medical students, each time they study a new disease. Overtired and overstressed – examining gravely ill patients in the wards, or their bottled remains in the laboratory – we found ourselves clutching our bodies in horror as symptoms seemed to leap out of the textbook page, and then into those terrified bodies. Symptoms of the latest disease spread regularly through the class like a virulent epidemic, the contagion blown swiftly among us by the wild Cape south-easter winds.

Hearing so often about the 'typical' symptoms of a disease, opens up the possibility of what's been called 'clinical mimicry'. It's a familiar feature of all medical practice, especially for the young, inexperienced doctor – a situation where the symptoms of one disease closely resemble those of another. Similar symptoms may be caused by very different diseases – or, as in Gary's case, by no disease at all.

Often labelled 'psychosomatic', this last group are seen as merely psychological (or 'functional') rather than physical (or 'organic').

Medical textbooks include many examples of such 'clinical mimicry', some with some underlying bodily disease, others not. They range from conditions such as *pseudo-gout* (which mimics real gout, but has a very different cause), to the more exotic *pseudocyesis* or 'pseudo-pregnancy' – a psychological condition where a woman, yearning to be pregnant, develops many of the symptoms of pregnancy, but without being actually pregnant. Some diseases, and their early symptoms, are more open to imitation than others. In the 19th century, because of their vague and varied presentations, both syphilis and tuberculosis were known to doctors as the 'great imitators'. Today it is heart disease, cancer and AIDS that generally fulfil that role.

In 1998, in the journal *Psychosomatic Medicine*, Elizabeth Miller reported from Japan on a mini-epidemic of another pseudo-disease – one that's been termed 'AIDS neurosis'. The first case was reported back in 1987, and many more have been reported since then. People with this syndrome usually have a variety of physical complaints, as well as depression, sleep disturbance, phobic tendencies, and suicidal ideas. And they all have the firm belief – despite all medical evidence to the contrary – that they are HIV positive. Most of the victims have been middle-aged men, feeling guilty about having had a sexual encounter with a foreign prostitute, and who have then misinterpreted any vague symptoms afterwards as evidence of AIDS. Miller quotes one AIDS counsellor as saying, '(The) Japanese are at much greater risk for developing AIDS neurosis than they are of getting AIDS.'

Meanwhile, from Britain, the USA and elsewhere, a growing number of cases of 'pseudo-AIDS' – also an unfounded, exaggerated fear of having contracted the disease – have also been reported. This happened especially during the early years of the epidemic, and especially in those who were already anxious or depressed.

Like the other 'great imitators', pseudo-angina has actually been around since long before Gary was born. It's been drifting out there for more than 150 years.

Back in 1854 a certain Dr William Stokes described the large group of 'nervous affections of the heart'. Such 'neurosis of the heart' might arise, he wrote, 'as in the case of hysteric disease, the accidental localisation of a wandering neurosis, which now affects one, and now another organ'. But he warned that sometimes they might well be accompanied by *real* physical disease.

It was Dr Walter Hayle Walshe of London who first coined the phrase 'pseudo-angina pectoris' in 1862, describing it as 'a form of complaint combining in a minor degree many of the characters of angina; and to this imitation of the true disease I propose to give the name of pseudo-angina'. His view was opposite to that of Dr Stokes, for he believed that 'genuine angina pectoris is undoubtedly a very rare affliction', and that it's 'pseudo' form was much more common.

'Its imitation is more common in males than females,' he noted, 'and in the higher than in the lower walks of society.'

Since then, many more 'nervous afflictions of the heart', with more exotic names attached to them, have been described – all of them precipitated by stress or exhaustion. During the US Civil War, psychosomatic chest pain, especially among Union soldiers, was known as 'Da Costa's syndrome', and then during the First World War as 'Soldier's Heart'. (By that war's end, 44, 000 British soldiers had been pensioned off with this diagnosis.) Later on it was known as 'Effort Syndrome', 'Cardiac Neurosis' or 'Neurocirculatory Aesthenia'. Like Drs Stokes and Walshe, a century earlier, Dr Paul Dudley White in 1951 wrote that these symptoms were likely to occur 'especially in hypersensitive individuals', or in those who were, 'weak, tired, sick, or nervous persons'. The treatment he prescribed included rest, reassurance and re-education, for he warned that otherwise the condition might result in 'days, weeks, or even years of invalid existence'.

Each year there seem to be more of these pseudo-diseases around. They are the unexpected by-product of the increasing diffusion of health information into the population – and especially of the stories told, on page or screen, of those who have suffered from certain diseases. And for their own reasons, and often completely unconsciously, some people, especially those who are stressed or exhausted, capture these stories, and make them their own. And then, in a sense, they *embody* them.

Others, such as the actor and the malingerer, do so more consciously. They become skilful practitioners of clinical mimicry. As are the sufferers from a group of odd conditions known to psychiatrists as 'somatoform disorders', which includes a number of the so-called 'factitious diseases'. People with these disorders deliberately distort the story of their symptoms, and produce misleading physical findings, sometimes actually inflicting the lesions on themselves. The most toxic form of this is 'Munchausen syndrome', also known as 'hospital addiction syndrome', named after that legendary teller of tall tales, Baron von Munchausen. These individuals often develop a detailed knowledge of medical matters, and a mastery of medical terminology. They travel from hospital to hospital, claiming to be gravely ill, and giving convincing accounts of the dramatic symptoms they are suffering from. Often this results in their undergoing unnecessary and expensive hospital tests, or even operations. They are known derisively as 'hospital hoboes'.

In the past, medical textbooks embroidered this group of 'factitious illnesses' with wonderfully colourful Latin names. Those hoping for an abdominal operation (a laparotomy) were said to have '*laparotimophilia migrans*'; those who claimed to be bleeding profusely from various parts of their body had '*haemorrhagica histrionica*'; those presenting with imaginary 'convulsions' had '*neurologica diabolica*'; a history of false 'heart attacks', atypical 'angina' or 'irregular heartbeats' meant '*cardiopathia fantastica*'; while patients who lied uncontrollably, giving fantastic and vivid descriptions of false events in their lives – such as the recent murder of close family members – probably had '*pseudologia fantastica*'.

The psychiatrist M Scott Peck has written that 'to name something correctly gives us a certain amount of power over it.' A key part of any doctor's task is to help this process along; to give a specific name – the diagnosis – to their patient's suffering, and thus to impose a sense of order onto chaos. But names misapplied can also be dangerous, especially diagnostic labels. In some serious diseases, such as cancer or heart disease, the power that resides in a name can rob them of hope, even lead other people to abandon them. In certain vulnerable people they can become a self-fulfilling prophecy. The name can take on its own dynamic. It can kill, as well as heal.

Another Monday morning, several weeks later. And afterwards, when I thought back on it, I recalled those other words of Dr William Stokes – the ones that, even today, still leave a bitter taste in my mouth.

Another man in his mid-40s sits across the desk from me, frowning with anxiety. Martin is complaining of several episodes of left chest pain that come and go, some general weakness, and an occasional shortness of breath. He, too, has been under stress lately, what with work and home-life, and some unexpected financial problems. And he also has three young children and a worried wife. As I listen to him, I am thinking to myself, 'What an amazing coincidence! How extraordinary the way these stories migrate so easily from person to person, like a San story carried on the wind, like a gust of contagion. And what's more, twice in such a short time!'

I examine Martin fully, and then reassure him. Except for a slightly raised blood pressure, I can find nothing wrong. But just to be quite sure, though I'm more relaxed now about his probable diagnosis, I refer him immediately to that same eminent cardiologist. A week or so later, a similar letter arrives. All the tests were negative. Once again, he writes to me, it seems to be a case of 'pseudo-angina'. He is just as surprised by the coincidence as I am.

On a Tuesday morning Martin and his wife come to see me to discuss the cardiologist's report. He is still rather tense, and still complaining of occasional chest pain, but, as with Gary, I reassure them that all the tests are OK; that the cardiologist thinks its just pseudo-angina from muscular spasms, due mainly to stress. It seems that Dr Stokes's 'wandering neurosis' has found yet another victim. The couple leave thanking me, grateful and relaxed, smiling at each other.

That Sunday in the early afternoon, Martin is sitting at the table in his dining room after a big lunch, his children playing in the next room, his wife sitting across from him – when suddenly he turns pale. He seems to be trying to tell her something, but the words never come out. Then he clutches his chest, and falls forward onto the table. The ambulance is called, the paramedics try their best to revive him. But it's too late to do anything.

When I hear the news, I am shocked. I telephone the cardiologist. My voice on the phone is husky and wavering, but shrill at the edges. 'But you *said* he didn't have angina,' I hear my voice rising. 'You *said* that the tests showed that he was OK. That he *didn't* have any heart trouble. That your tests are 95 per cent accurate'.

For a moment there is silence. Then his voice on the line is calm, solicitous, as if talking to a hysterical child. As if he were having to repeat a story to it for the hundredth time, in order to make it understand. 'Yes, but as I explained to you last time,' he says, 'they *are* 95 per cent accurate 95 per cent. It's tragic, I agree, but what can one say? He just must have been one of the other 5 per cent'.

I notice his voice on the phone has also risen in volume, and that his breathing has become rapid and noisy, almost as if he were hyperventilating. I feel the quick gusts of a powerful wind whistling over the line towards me, blowing the words right out of my mouth, and then scattering them into the air.

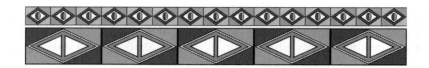

CHAPTER 5

MASKS OF SKIN

According to my dermatology textbook – its glossy pages filled with bright colour-photographs of rashes, warts, bumps, blemishes and moles – 'The skin is an extensive organ covering the exterior of the body.' Its most important function, it says, 'is to serve as a barrier between the individual and the external environment'. It describes in detail the two main layers of the skin: the outer, visible 'epidermis', made up of specialised cells known as 'stratified squamous epithelium'; and the 'dermis', a complex and irregular layer of different types of cells and receptors that lies beneath it, and which acts as both its support and nourishment, like the foundations and energy supply of an extensive building.

The book then goes on to describe how the skin is not only the largest organ of the body, accounting for about 15 per cent of the total body weight, but is also one of its most important. It envelopes and protects the body, but is also a vital source of sensation, insulation and temperature control. And yet this cool, scientific description of the skin is not the whole story. As the outer capsule of the human sense of self, it is much more than that. And it often has its own story to tell.

For Mary in particular, it's a fragile parchment on which she has inscribed, in a series of pictograms, a message to the world. And to herself.

It's always difficult to estimate her age, for she's a shadowy, rather colourless figure, who blends easily into the darker parts of any room that she enters. Sometimes she seems almost invisible. Seating herself across the desk from me, she speaks softly, almost inaudibly. The clothes that she wears are mostly a faded black or a dullish grey. Even her face seems faded – its cheeks bleached and gaunt, her cheekbones half in shadow. Her hair, like thin strands of liquorice, is lustreless and streaked with grey.

Today she is complaining of a pain, sharp and gripping, in the lower part of her abdomen.

I take down the full story of the pain, carefully writing it into her medical records: when it began, under what circumstances, and exactly where. Also, what makes it any better or worse, and how it's developed since it began. But when I ask her to lie down on my examination couch so that I can examine her, she seems reluctant, oddly hesitant. For a moment her eyes flicker from me to the door, then back again. Then she pulls her grey jacket closely around her thin shoulders, and slowly rises from her chair.

As she climbs onto the examination couch, behind the rattan screen, and lies herself down, she seems to shrink from the bright angled light mounted above it. Then with a sudden jerk, like a painter unveiling her latest work, she pulls up all her clothing.

For a moment I catch my breath. My hands, moving forward to examine her, pause in mid-air. I have never seen anything like this before.

It is not only those elaborate Celtic knots and spirals that circle her breasts. Nor all those spiky Chinese pictographs that decorate her upper trunk. It is rather how the skin of her chest and abdomen, and the pale skin of her flanks, has now been revealed as a multi-coloured garden filled with mythological creature. In the cold fluorescent light of my consulting room, her skin surface is a proud display of blue, green, red and yellow creatures, each one rapidly expanding in size, then shrinking again, with every anxious breath she takes. There are several gryphons there, an eagle, a sort of mermaid, and those two large oriental dragons that rear up on either side of her body. With jagged wings and tails and sharp white teeth, they are blowing sharp coils of wild red fire out of their greenish jaws, the flames flickering up towards her nipples, each one pierced by a tiny silver ring. Both dragons are rising right out of the depths of her groin as if they'd just been born there. They are flying up to meet a cascade of tiny scarlet roses, crucifixes, pierced hearts, and butterflies (of many different colours) that are flowing down towards them. Mingled among them, I spot a flock of minute birds swooping down from her upper chest towards her sternum, fluttering their wings between her breasts, and circling her umbilicus. And there is more. On her arms, hidden by her long dark sleeves, I see a line of small rococo scrolls, like battle honours on a regimental flag. Some of the names within them seem to have been crudely removed, the skin still raw and unfinished, while others have been turned into palimpsests, with new names tattooed carefully over the old.

Gently probing the wings and body of one dragon, and then the other, palpating a gryphon or two, I can find no tenderness, no swellings, no signs of inner inflammation. Her abdomen seems to be normal, the pain probably due only to a cramp, one that will respond easily to a pain-killer or an anti-spasmodic. And yet, there is another type of tenderness here, another deep type of pain. For it is clear that Mary's body is telling a particular story, though as yet I cannot decode the complex language in which it is written.

Seeing this aspect of her for the first time, I assume that her skin is an expression of her inner life: decorative, exuberant, proud, and filled with multiple colours, movement and aesthetic form. I wonder for a moment whether, like the San – the indigenous people of South Africa – her inner and outer stories are somehow continuous with one another, or else closely related. For the San believed that the painted surface of their beautiful cave paintings was only the outer membrane of the story that they represented. And that the events portrayed there (a shaman's dance, a hunt, a herd of kudu) all continued deep into the interior of the rock behind it. But later I learn that I am wrong.

And then I meet Janet. She's been recently discharged from hospital and is, I am told, one of those rare cases of Munchausen's syndrome – a classic 'hospital addict'. One of those sad or mad people, addicted to surgical operations, and to the focused attention that they can bring. Over the years she has had numerous, unnecessary operations on different parts of her body. Mystified by her bizarre and ambiguous symptoms, a succession of surgeons have operated on her gall bladder, her appendix, tonsils, breasts and womb. Others have remodelled her nose and ears, and removed numerous wrinkles, warts and blemishes from her skin. Each time it is as though some *incubus*, some small repository of evil, has somehow settled in one part of her body, and then caused all the problems in her life. It can only be exorcised by an operation, a willing sacrifice of that part of her body to the dark gods of her psyche.

After years of repeated surgery, the surface of Janet's skin, criss-crossed by scars, has become the visual record of a much deeper anguish. When I examine her in my consulting room, it reminds me of the annotated map of a battlefield, still marked by abandoned trenches and long strands of rusty barbed wire. Here, too, a certain message is on display. Not of a garden of mythological creatures enveloping and protecting its owner, but rather one of war, pain and ritual sacrifice. The differences between her skin surface and Mary's are those between a ruined landscape and an art museum. And yet, as I realise later, Janet's text is the more consistent of the two. Like those cave paintings of the San, her inner and outer stories bear a much greater resemblance to one another.

Stretched out on the examination couch, her body surface, repeatedly violated by scalpels and probes, reminds me for some reason of Franz Kafka's story *In the Penal Colony*. In that story, the punishment for breaking one of the Colony's laws is to have that same law tattooed all over one's body surface. The sentence is carried out by a complex machine – a diabolical device of levers, cogs and sharp needles that inscribes the words deep into the skin. But unlike any ordinary tattoo, the text doesn't end at the surface, for the needles inscribe it so deeply that they penetrate into the body's interior, and eventually destroy it. Much like Janet's operation scars, the act of inscribing the text becomes a form of punishment in itself. The wounds decorate the public parts of the body but, like a San rock painting, they also continue deep into its interior.

Such wounds, whether from surgery or tattooing, can be seen as a type of closure, a way of reclaiming the body for oneself. As the anthropologist Susan Benson has put it, 'The emphasis is upon the marked skin as a defence or seal against its own past, while the violence and pain entailed in the process of cutting or piercing both mimics and expunges a previous violation.' Tattoos are thus 'scars that speak' – but they do not necessarily demand a reply. They are wounds whose aim is to heal a much deeper wound.

It is only many years later, in fact, after I have moved on to another job elsewhere, that I meet someone who tells me Mary's other story. The one that she has always held deep within herself, never revealing it to me, or to any of her other doctors. It's her personal history, always kept carefully concealed inside its decorated envelope of skin. It's the story of a chaotic childhood, of violence, abuse and terror. A narrative of how she and her sisters were abused, again and again, by a series of drunken 'uncles' that her mother took into their house, in different parts of the country. The mother was tiny and terrified, often drunk herself, and could never protect her. Later Mary abused her own body even more with different types of drugs, injecting them slowly into her veins and skin like a careful nurse. There were also several abortions, drunken boyfriends, and an arrest or two. She has never had children.

It's a story very different from the vivid, colourful glory of the mythological garden on her surface, filled with beauty, life and gentle movement.

In her book *Skin*, Claudia Benthien points out that the words 'shame' and 'skin' have the same Indo-Germanic root, meaning 'to cover', and that the two concepts are closely related. For above all the skin is the covering of the nakedness of the inner body, a barrier against shame, a protection from enquiring eyes.

In most European languages, 'skin' has actually got two very different meanings. And I have encountered both of them, in my time at the Medical Centre. One is as the protective cover, something that encloses and conceals the Self, but is something other than 'the Self'. Susan Benson writes how, in this view, the skin is only the outer capsule of the person, the boundary between them and other people. 'Personhood' is conceived of in terms of what lies deep 'inside' in some ethereal, authentic 'essence' of self. So the body's surface becomes merely a blank parchment on which this inner self can express itself, and on which it can inscribe a variety of different messages, from religious images to personal symbols. It becomes a site for self-presentation and personal creativity. It can be clothed, painted, perfumed, tattooed, pierced, cut, scarified or circumcised, or else altered endlessly by cosmetic surgery. Each of these is a 'statement of the self', displayed on the skin for all to see. The difference between self and skin becomes that between inner essence and outer appearance. Even beauty can only be 'skin deep'.

In the second, the skin itself stands for the whole person. It actually *is* the person, the representation of the whole. In a sense you *are* your skin, for it's a public display of who you really are, both within and without. Your identity, your place in the world, and your relationships with other people. Even your inner life. In the South Seas, where bodily and facial tattoos are common (the word comes from the Polynesian *tatau*), Benson writes that 'it is on the skin that personhood is located.' For the Maoris and others in that area, tattoos can be a complex visual code, as well as a form of spiritual armour. They are a public declaration of who they are: a display of their status or occupation, their identity as a warrior or a member of a particular group or family. In parts of Africa, too, skin markings, such as facial scarification, can also act as a visual map of kinship and ancestry, a fixed, immutable display of personal identity.

Although tattooing is now common in the West, it's a relatively recent practice. It was brought to Europe and North America only in the 18th and 19th centuries by sailors who'd learned the skill from visits to the South Sea islands. In the early days, only those sailors and soldiers regularly tattooed their bodies. It's only since the 1960s, and the so-called 'Tattoo Renaissance', that tattooing has moved from the marginal to the mainstream: from working-class convicts, prostitutes, street gangs, bikers, circus 'freaks' and performers to middle-class followers of radical protest movements or of New Age philosophy. For both men and women, being tattooed has become an expression of autonomy, power and self-reclamation.

Many of the neo-tribalists of today's urban jungle wear tattoos based on Chinese, Japanese, Native American, African or Hawaiian designs. Inscribing them onto their skins can be seen as a way of acting out, in a symbolic sense, the themes of the natural, the pure, the primitive, the mythological – in opposition to the shallow values, anomie and polluted chaos of modern urban life.

Mrs N is obsessed with her skin, but in a very different way. And yet her choice of obsession is both contemporary and up to date. She is a businesswoman in a shiny black trouser suit, with shiny black high-heeled shoes and a white frilly blouse. She is middle-40s and middle-class, divorced, with a carefully sprayed hairdo, tiny gold earrings and a double row of pearls. Her make-up is flawless. On one wrist she wears a thin gold bracelet, on the other a small golden watch at which she glances nervously every few minutes. Under one arm she usually carries a shiny black handbag, with a glittering gold clasp. She seems to be always in a hurry, always rushing between appointments.

Whenever I have visited her house when she's been ill, I've been struck by its exaggerated neatness, glimpsing my puzzled reflection in the shiny surfaces and spotless mirrors in room after room, and by the brittle, breakable atmosphere that seems to accompany them. And struck, too, by her glistening kitchen, and the sparkling varnish of her dinner table; and the gleaming glass shelves of her sideboard, as clear as water, crowded with crystal ornaments and tiny figurines. And I am also struck by her excessive anxiety about the tiniest spill on a carpet, a stain on a tablecloth, or some minor mark on the furniture or on the pure white walls that encase her on all sides – as well as by the tiniest imperfection of her skin.

At the Medical Centre she seems to spend hours across the desk from me, pointing out to me this faint blemish, or that minute mark, tiny bump or irregular area on her skin surface, most of which I can hardly see. For that is where all Mrs N's anxiety seems to have settled – on that pale, fragile boundary between her over-anxious self and the threatening world around her. Over the years this anxiety has marked her body surface deeply, like an invisible tattoo. It has turned it into an eternally vulnerable membrane whose surface must be regularly soothed and reassured – by creams, ointments, liniments and lotions, by expensive laser and depilation treatments, and by the veritable alchemist's laboratory of soap, scent and deodorant bottles that she keeps in her shining, immaculate bathroom. It must be kept under constant surveillance, endlessly re-checked for any imperfection that might herald the decline of its protective function.

In a further cruel twist, each time she's feeing stressed or embarrassed, or finds herself walking in a chill wind, her unreliable boundary lets her down. She breaks out in a red, blotchy, itchy rash that rises up her neck in angry flames from below her silken blouse, like an extensive tattoo, inscribed in scarlet ink.

Mrs N appears to live her life in constant terror of some dirt or disorder breaking the neat symmetry of her suburban life, disrupting the symbolic boundaries that she has so carefully erected – both at home and at work – between herself and the chaotic, dangerous world around her. It seems to be a life where every surface, but most especially her skin, is inherently unreliable – a site of potential danger, of pollution or penetration.

Mrs N seems to be an example of the very contemporary phenomenon, one that Jonathan Marshall terms 'boundary anxiety'. He sees it as a new and profound anxiety, a major issue in Western industrial society. For in our post-modernist world of rapid movement and rapid social change, personal identity is no longer as fixed as it once was. It has become increasingly fluid and changeable, and seemingly unstable.

Bombarded by the seductive messages of consumer society, many people now define themselves by the endless series of temporary, false selves created by advertising and the media, by the endless consumption of new goods and new lifestyles, and by fads and fashions that change every year. And also, says Marshall, the boundaries between groups of people, and the methods of maintaining those boundaries, seem increasingly insecure and a focus of anxiety. Previously firm boundaries, such as those against out-groups like foreigners or immigrants or those of a different social class, now appear to be breaking down, and so are the more intimate boundaries between self and others, men and women, work and home, 'us' and 'them', inside and outside. In fact, many of these boundaries – these symbolic 'skins' – are what for most people in previous generations helped to define 'a person'.

In her *Theatres of the Body*, the psychoanalyst Joyce McDougall has described the similar, but very extreme, case of Georgette, one of her clients, someone who at times 'did not truly distinguish between my body and hers, nor between our personal identities'. Georgette, too, had difficulty in experiencing her skin as the firm, impenetrable boundary of her Self. One year, when McDougall came back tanned from her vacation, Georgette cried out in horror, 'What have you done to *my* face? My face is hurting badly.' And each time McDougall went away on vacation, Georgette broke out in a red, raw rash all over her body. It's almost as if she'd been 'flayed alive'. 'As though,' writes McDougall, 'with each separation her epidermis was torn away from mine'. She calls this situation, 'one body for two'. Georgette may be only a single case, and an extreme example at that, of someone without a firmly defined body boundary. But perhaps she – together with both Mary and Mrs N – are emblematic of another very modern condition: the terror, and sense of vulnerability, of the *skinless self*.

The year 1543 was an important landmark in the history of anatomy, and the history of skin. In that year the first great European textbook of anatomy appeared, that prize of dissection art, the *De Humani Corporis Fabrica* of Andreas Vesalius. Significantly, it was also a book from which the human skin had disappeared almost completely. Among the 300 detailed illustrations are full-page woodcuts of skinless 'muscle men' – human figures stripped down to an elaborate underwear of muscles, ligaments, tendons and bones. Like actors on a stage, or mannequins on a catwalk, these skinless bodies strut or pose across the pages in a variety of settings, their bodies raw, naked, exposed. Some adopt affected poses among classical tableaux of rocks, trees or picturesque ruins. Others hang from gallows, their limbs splayed to show the muscles and ligaments of the limbs and trunk. A number of full-page woodcuts show complete adult skeletons, also arranged in lifelike postures. These collages of bones seem alive, and many appear to be sad or contemplative. One skeleton leans in a Hamlet pose over a marble tomb, his tibias and fibulas crossed, holding a solitary skull in his bony fingers, with his facial bones arranged in a thoughtful look.

The *De Humani Corporis Fabrica* is a predecessor to Günter von Hagen's *Körperwelten* ('Body Worlds') exhibition, seen by millions since 1995, with its display of 'plastinated' corpses, also quite skinless and reduced mainly to their muscles and bones. As in Vesalius, these figures are arranged in tableaux of lifelike poses: a basketball player, an archer, a swimmer, an equestrian. One figure, the 'Skin Man', actually holds aloft his flayed skin like a discarded set of old clothes.

But 1543, when Vesalius's great work appeared, was, by an ironic coincidence, the same year in which Copernicus published his *De Revolutionibus Orbium Celestium*, in which he argued that the earth revolved around the sun, and not the other way round. Copernicus's heliocentric view places our planet not at the centre, but right at the periphery of the solar system. Vesalius, by contrast, places the human body at the very centre of the landscape, the core of his universe. But he portrays it stripped of its protective, individualised mask of skin, down to its muscles and ligaments, even to its core of bones.

It's a very prophetic picture. For Vesalius's skinless bodies can be seen as a precognition of a very contemporary phenomenon – the growing sense of permeability, and irrelevance, of the skin itself. It is a development to which medicine itself has contributed – making the human body, for the first time, almost transparent to the naked eye, with the aid of its X-rays, its scans and its probes. What was once hidden inside, is now exposed to view, and in the process the skin is dissolved, making it seem almost invisible.

In the past, medicine has had an uneven attitude towards the body's surface. Before the Enlightenment, it was perceived as porous and open, and in constant connection with the world around it. The skin surface was, in Claudia Benthien's words, 'a place of permeability and mysterious metamorphoses', with 'a multitude of possible openings'. Based on the theories of Galen, European medicine at that time saw illness as the outer expression of some inner disharmony, usually an imbalance of the four *humours* of the body (blood, phlegm, black bile, yellow bile). These were waste products created by the breakdown of food and drink, and to maintain health they had to be regularly removed from the body. They oozed out of it in the form of sweat, saliva, urine, stools, semen, menstrual blood or 'vapours', and nothing should block or delay this constant flow. In illness, the aim of the physician was to 'draw' these excess humours out of the patient as quickly as possible, 'evacuating' them with the aid of enemas, emetics, gargles, massages, hot baths and inhalations. Many 'evacuations' could only be done via the skin – by bloodletting, cupping, leaches, scarification, sweating, blistering, or the application of special poultices.

The body then was not yet the sealed container for the individualised self (what Alan Watts later called the 'skin-encapsulated ego') that it eventually became. Only from the Enlightenment onwards, with the growth of individualism, did it become seen as an entity surrounded by its own capsule, a boundary of smooth impenetrable skin. 'Body' and 'self' then became virtually the same thing, both occupying the same space, both bounded by the same epidermis. Disease was now due to penetration of this little island of flesh by some external agent, such as a germ or virus, especially via one of its orifices – rather than to some humoural imbalance within. The interior of the sealed body was hidden from view; mysterious and invisible.

But then along came X-rays and scans, and the importance of the skin dissolved yet again.

With skin and self so closely connected, for some it has become important that their visible body should be malleable, and capable of endless improvement. They will tattoo it or paint it or otherwise adorn it, while for those who can afford it, cosmetic surgery now offers the best chance of radically sculpting their body's surface into a different form – even if, despite their fervent wish, it cannot do the same for the personality enclosed within it.

In 2003 the journal *New Scientist* reported that surgeons in the USA had carried out no less than 1.8 million cosmetic operations that year, the largest number ever recorded, and nearly double the figures for 1997. They included facelifts, rhinoplasties ('nose jobs'), breast implants, liposuction, tummy tucks, brow lifts, hair implants, laser hair removal and cosmetic dentistry, as well as more temporary measures, like Botox injections, and the use of false teeth, eyelashes and fingernails. Some surgeons carried out more drastic, intimate operations, to meet the growing demand for surgical remodelling of the female external genitalia, to make them conform to the 'ideal' images commonly seen in pornographic films and magazines. In contrast, restoration of the hymen (hymenoplasty) is now common in some communities, in order to restore a semblance of 'virginity' before marriage.

All this means that the skin has become more than just a blank canvas, awaiting the tattooist's needle or the beautician's brush. Nor is it any longer as immutable as it once was. It has become clay, ready to be moulded into different forms by the gloved hands and scalpels of the cosmetic surgeon – that highly trained, highly paid, sculptor of living flesh.

All visible alterations to the skin's surface – whether by tattoos, scars, layers of make-up, or the sculpturing of a cosmetic surgeon – can turn it into a type of mask, though one attached permanently to the body. And like all masks, a mask of skin can both conceal and reveal at the same time. It can obscure the individual, but can also release some inner, uninhibited self hidden somewhere deep within. The Jungian analyst Aniela Jaffé has written how in psychological terms, while individual identity is submerged by a mask, at the same time that mask also 'transforms its wearer into an archetypal image'. She sees, for example, the animal masks worn in tribal initiation rituals as revealing the archetypal 'animal-being' within, the one 'which lives in him as his instinctual psyche' – as it does within all of us. The ritual itself acts as a way of acknowledging, integrating, and controlling these primitive 'animal' impulses. Different types of mask will reveal different types of archetypal identity, such as the trickster (the clown or the harlequin), the hero (Batman, Spiderman, Zorro, or the *luchadores*, the masked wrestlers of Mexico), or even the villain (the terrorist, the robber, the highwayman). Wearing a mask may conceal individual identity, but at the same time it can re-establish it as a 'fixed type' – whether a psychological archetype, a creature from mythology, or as one of the characters of the *Commedia dell'arte*.

For some people, the intimate masks of skin can become one way of 'fixing' their individual identity: of making it – at least on the surface – seem permanent and firm. Like many other masks, they can be seen as an attempt to free the person from the usual constraints of time, condensing past, present and future, and blurring them all together into a numinous sense of timelessness, of time-out-of-time. The mask becomes an antidote to the passage of time, and to the anxiety caused by aging and decline, and the endless change and instability inherent in all human life.

Above all, those masks of skin can be a strategy for dealing with the growing existential terror of the 'skinless self' – naked and vulnerable in the harsh, Brave New World of today.

Medical practice has taught me one bitter lesson, over and over again. That some wounds can simply never be healed. Despair and grief cannot always be kept indefinitely at bay. Not by tattoos, nor by any other mask of skin.

Many years after my first sight of Mary's skin, I happen to meet someone who tells me what has happened to her in the years since I last encountered her. It's an upsetting story, for it seems that after a long period of relative stability, she returned to using drugs heavily again, and for a while was living in a chaotic household with yet another drunken, abusive boyfriend. Gradually her health began to decline. She became chronically ill, lost weight steadily, and was soon on her way to an early death. It seems that her mask of skin could not protect her after all. It had been fatally penetrated, both from within and from without.

From what that person told me, I imagined that in those last years in the mythological garden, the gryphons and dragons and other beasts had all run wild. They had torn down its walls, gnawed away at its foliage, and set the flowers on fire. The garden itself had fallen into ruin. The eagle and the little birds had become shrunken and limp, and had hardly ever flown. Until finally one day – and not so long ago – on the pale and wrinkled floor of the garden, punctured by scabs and scars and the infected marks of many needles, the whole flock of brightly coloured butterflies had suddenly stopped flying, their wings lying faded and still.

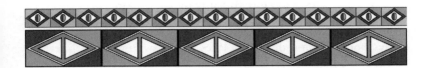

CHAPTER
6

WAITING FOR GODETTE

Once upon a time...' they usually begin, or sometimes, 'In the beginning...'. They are Myths of Origin, creation myths. The oldest stories of all. The story of the birth of the world, or of the true origins of this fact or that. And yet Jonathan doesn't ever use either of those phrases. He tells his story in a different way. He is a thin, worried young man, with round rimless glasses and a wispy beard, and as he speaks his pale, delicate forehead becomes corrugated with frowns.

Another day, another long procession of stories passing through my consulting room. Tales of pain or anxiety, stories of suffering. One story-teller after another sitting across the desk from me. For medicine is all about stories, or rather it should be. A place to share those stories with another person, to mingle the patients' own stories with those of the doctor, and – with a sense of relief – to go home with something new.

When he was a child, Jonathan tells me, his family were expatriates in a certain hot, dusty country in Africa. His father was a senior executive there in a large multi-national company. They lived in an enclave of other wealthy expatriates, in big houses, each with its own corps of servants, its own large swimming pool fringed with palm trees.

One day, when he is about five or six, his father takes him to their swimming pool to teach him how to swim. His mother isn't there that day. Perhaps she is in another of her depressions, or maybe secretly drinking again. From what Jonathan tells me, he was always a nervous, highly strung child, and that day he is particularly anxious. Water has

49

always worried him – the ocean, lakes, rivers, swimming pools, even a village pond. He much prefers solid hills and fields, even the dusty sweep of the desert outside of town.

That day, in his new, tight swimming costume, with the midday sun beating down on him, the boy feels particularly nervous.

They reached the edge of the pool, and he stands staring down at its rippling surface, and at the blue shifting tiles so far below. 'Jump!' says his father. 'Don't worry, Jonny, just jump in and I'll jump in too, to support you in the water – and then I'll teach you how to swim.'

The boy jumps in. The water feels icy, a sudden shock to his pale little body. He feels it closing over his head. With panic he feels himself sinking down, struggling and kicking, to the very bottom of the pool. He cannot breathe, he cannot swim. Part of him is still waiting for his father to jump in and save him, but nothing happens. Nothing. No father, and no rescue. He is alone, abandoned in the water, and beginning to die. The world around him is blue and chill, and beginning to blur. He sinks deeper and deeper, swallowing water, arms flailing, kicking out. Still no father appears. It feels like he is almost dead, drowned in the pool, when he suddenly feels his father's strong hands gripping him, pulling him, then raising him to the surface of the pool. He is spluttering, retching, sobbing. His father looks at him with pity, mixed with contempt. 'OK, OK,' he says, 'Just relax now. No need to make such a fuss. No need to cry like that. You've got to learn how to swim the hard way. Got to learn to be a man. '

For days afterwards, Jonathan is hysterical, inconsolable. He never swims in that pool again.

Years pass. The boy becomes a man, but still he refers back to that particular incident. It's a story that he often tells; sometimes to himself, sometimes to other people. Sometimes to a doctor. It has become the lens through which he views all the negative experiences of his life, gathering them together into a single pattern, a single image. It helps him explain to himself his fraught relationships with his boss (the one who makes him feel helpless, vulnerable), his wife (the one who never listens to him, especially when he's ill or upset), his brother (the one who always lets him down), his friend (the one who never returns his phone calls), and even his neighbour (the noisy one, whose music keeps him awake at night, despite his complaints). And, of course, it explains his relationship with his father, now elderly and frail.

Years later, back in Britain, in one workplace and relationship after another, he recounts how he sometimes still feels the icy blue waters closing over his head. He gasps, splutters, feels himself sinking helplessly and struggling, nearing death. Sometimes, especially in confrontations with his boss, he finds he can hardly breathe, and begins to pant and to gasp. For many years, every workplace became a swimming pool, every relationship a type of drowning.

Over the years, the story has been fashioned, and re-fashioned, by a series of psychotherapists that he's seen. He has even undergone psychoanalysis for a time, lying on a couch for year after year. At great expense, each type of therapist that he's seen has helped him to refine, and develop, that explanatory story, till its current version feels almost perfect to him.

But not quite perfect enough. For he tells me how, over several years, his latest therapist has gently dismantled that central swimming pool myth – the story that he has always used to explain so much in his life, and especially the birth and persistence of his unhappiness. It is not so much a *creatio ex nihilo* (creation out of nothing), but rather a story that builds on other stories, on prior emotional themes within his own history, and that of his particular family.

Instead, over time, two more specialised myths have gradually taken their place, each one emerging from those regular, intense discussions with the therapist. One of them (the swimming pool story) he still uses to explain his fraught relationship with his boss, and with the other male authority figures in his life. The other one (his mother's passive compliance in the swimming pool incident) he applies mainly to his uneasy relationships with women. It's like a type of meiosis, or cell division, but for Jonathan it's the beginning of emotional growth. Much later, I am hopeful, these two will split again into smaller, more specialised myths. Into four then, and maybe even more.

My anthropology studies taught me that a *myth* is more than just a story. It's much more than mere fiction or untruth, for to those who believe in it, that myth is totally true.

A myth is usually a tale that originates in the dim past, but it always has a special function – to explain how everything began, and why things are as they are today. In cultures and communities throughout the world, myths, like the *Just So* stories of Rudyard Kipling ('How the Leopard got his Spots', 'How the Camel got his Hump'), explain how the world came to be as it is. Whether historically true or not, these stories – like Jonathan's own personal myth – are used not only to explain the present, but also to justify it.

Creation myths are the best-known form. They are found, it seems, in every human society. And interestingly, many of them share common themes with one another. Whether they are religious or scientific, whether you believe in Genesis or the Big Bang theory, these stories are all about how the world began: the formation of reality, how it was done, and perhaps Who created it. 'In the beginning...' always produces a very special type of narrative. One that usually begins with a sense of a primal chaos or formlessness, but is then followed by the dramatic arrival of order and meaning. This symbolic point sometimes marks the birth of the Universe, or of the First Man or First Woman, the very first Animals and Birds, or the origins of Good and Evil, Light and Darkness, Time and Space. Some stories, like that of the Garden of Eden, are all about the beginnings of self-awareness and personal responsibility, as well as of the loss of innocence, the discovery of sexual shame. Others, especially in agrarian communities, are more cyclical, and retelling at every winter, spring and harvest festival celebrates the annual death and rebirth of the earth itself, and of all the plants, crops and rivers that live within it.

Medicine, too, has its own myths of origin and development. Almost every book on medical history tells the same story: one of inexorable progress from superstition to science, from darkness to light. Usually they begin with a description of the bizarre beliefs, odd theories and useless treatments of past generations of physicians – and then take the story triumphantly up to the fluorescent-lit hospitals of today, with all their wonder drugs, surgical miracles and glittering diagnostic machines.

But actual medical practice is about a more intimate type of myth. Often it's another type of myth of origin, such as the personal myths of people like Jonathan – and each one of us has our own, individual version of it. It's the narrative usually of the more painful experiences of our life, and how they all began. It situates the individual's life at the centre of a personal cosmos, somewhere between the Beginning of the world and its End. Most of these personal myths are self-crafted, but others have been created with the help of family or friends, or of doctors and therapists – those great myth-makers of the modern world. Often a consultation with either of these professionals has some resemblance to a creative writing class, a setting in which the participants' own stories of suffering can be endlessly re-fashioned, and re-edited, over weeks or even years, with new elements being regularly added, and others allowed to fall away. In psychotherapy particularly, therapist and client often work together not only to improve the client's symptoms, but also to develop a convincing narrative, a myth of creation for that individual. One that answers the question, 'Why have things gone wrong in my life?' At the end of the therapy, it will become a special gift from therapist to client, one that the client will carry away with him or her: the gift of narrative. A story that that person can use to explain events, perhaps for the rest of his or her life. Like Jonathan's swimming pool story, a 'Just So' story, tailored especially for him.

In certain ways, a personal myth may resemble the type of creation myths of nations, tribes or religious groups described by anthropologists. Often it, too, is a tale of difficult beginnings, of deep wounds, betrayals and battles, of harsh tests of endurance and faith, and eventually of triumph. Frequently it has a similar cast of characters to many of those communal myths, from powerful heroes, heroines and villains, to kings and queens, monsters and tricksters. And all of this is woven together into the story of an epic struggle, from childhood onwards, to overcome great obstacles – both within the individual's psyche, and in the world outside. And having overcome them, and survived, the hero or heroine often emerges from the struggle with a greater wisdom, having found the hidden treasure. The one that we now call '*insight*'.

For Jungians, there is a different type of resemblance between the personalised myths of an individual's life, and those cosmogenic myths that tell of the origin and development of the universe itself. As David Maclagan describes in his book *Creation Myths*, 'every person's life is, consciously or unconsciously, a creative evolution,' and a vital aspect of this process is the growth of *individuation* – marked by the separation of ego from non-ego, consciousness from unconsciousness. He sees this process as the psychological equivalent of 'such cosmogonic scenes as the separation of light from darkness or the parting of Father Sky from Mother Earth'. Thus in many mythologies there is a 'parallel between the pattern of individual life-processes and that of creation as a whole'. 'In the beginning...' can therefore be either the story of one's personal genesis and development, or that of the world itself.

In order to keep their power alive, myths need to be repeatedly told or acted out, often in a public and ritualised form. The performance is not only a way of reminding the spectators of the myth's importance, but also of re-creating each time the basic world-view of those who take part – and in this way, helping to carry it forward into the next generation.

The psychiatrist John Byng-Hall has described the power of one particular communal myth that intimately affects the individual. It is known as the 'family myth' or 'family script'. This usually consists of a set of stories and subliminal messages that are passed down within a family, from generation to generation. All families have them, in one form or another. Often they are designed to guide and protect the members of the family by telling them which roles they must adopt, how to interact with one another, and how to deal with the world outside. Within each family these stories are 'woven into the tapestry of self-perception and self-deception'. They become a way of both constructing reality, and providing a blueprint for how to deal with it. And yet for all their power, most people are not aware of the family myths that they have inherited, the ones that secretly control so much of their lives. '[These] myths are elusive,' writes Byng-Hall, 'now you see them: now you don't. It is easier to see someone else's than one's own.'

Family myths are a bit like theatre, where each member of the cast has a copy of the script, and each person plays a different role within the same play. Just like the legends handed down in tribal societies, they are stories about the family and the world, and how they came to be that way. They tell the family members how they should behave to one another, and to the outside world. They help ensure that the family's world-view continues, carrying it forward from one generation to the next. 'Within each telling of the story,' says Byng-Hall, 'the current rules of the family are encoded.'

Like the ritual re-enactment of a tribal myth, retelling the family story – or acting it out in real life – is a way of ensuring that the world of the family continues, just as it was before. That tomorrow is very similar to yesterday – and also to the day before that.

'You're a good listener,' says the man. 'You must be a priest or a doctor. You're not a therapist, I hope?'

I glance out through the train windows. The late afternoon landscape is whizzing past, a blur of trees, hills, suburbs and tiny stations, the train snaking past them and into the countryside, speeding on its way. There are several more hours of the journey to go, and the person sitting across from me – who introduces himself as Larry – is plump and in his mid-40s, with a florid distracted face.

There is no escape. I have no choice, but to nod sympathetically now and again, sometimes to smile or to frown, and always to try to keep up eye contact with him, however tired I may feel. He pours himself some more tea from the pot, then some into my cup. As I sip at the tepid liquid and munch on the dry, tasteless biscuits that accompany them, he settles himself back and begins his story. He says, with a smile, that he's trapped inside it. He cannot ever abandon it. As he speaks, I soon recognise it as one of those personal myths of suffering, the ones I so often encounter in medical practice. But this one sounds particularly fluent and well rehearsed, almost as if, like the Ancient Mariner, he has already told it many times, and to many other strangers that he's met along the way.

It soon becomes clear that Larry is still pre-Copernican. For he seems to see himself at the very centre of the universe, and every other person orbits about him. In that sense he has not yet heard Galileo's message – even though it's centuries old – that the earth is *not* the centre of our universe, but rather at its periphery. And possibly, he may never do so.

His own personal myth, as he tells it, sounds dangerous and destructive. As the remainder of the day rushes past, and the twilight thickens outside, he describes it to me with frequent frowns and an occasional wry smile. It seems to illustrate, once again, the power of a mythic story over a particular human life. But unlike Jonathan's, it's a myth of the future, rather than one of the past. It's the image of a magical World-to-Come, not of a long-lost Garden of Eden. Larry says that over the years, it has caused him much heartache.

His story sounds very different from those personal stories that can prove so useful or creative, especially for believers, mystics or writers. For in their hands these same stories of suffering are allowed to develop, often over many years, into something really beautiful, often a great work of art, or a great religious idea, like a story of redemption or enlightenment. Like a pearl formed in an oyster by a grit of pain, they can emerge one day as a beautiful, perfectly rounded shape, a luminous jewel to be worn and displayed to others.

But Larry's tale is more like a Moebius Ring (a surface that is non-orientable), with him travelling round and round it like a speeding train, but never really getting anywhere. It appears to have dominated his life up to this very moment. Listening to his description, in sharp, sometimes painful detail, I have to fight to stay awake. My eyes are beginning to cloud over, a storm cloud of headaches is gathering inside my head.

For it's all about his lifetime wait, and his relentless search, for the perfect woman. The one that his parents (sitting on the settee, holding hands, smiling at one another) had always told him to find and then to marry. The one they always referred to as 'the right woman'.

All his life Larry has searched for Her. He tells me how he has searched across cities and continents, through clubs and pubs and many different social gatherings. He has searched through the internet, the newspapers, and the dating adverts in many magazines. But still, he says, he's not yet found her. He has been on one date after another. Each time he thinks he's found someone, his parents have taken him aside and shaken their heads. 'She's very nice,' they say. 'She really is. But for you, she's definitely not the right woman.' And each time he finds himself agreeing with them, and usually with some relief. Looking at her more closely now, he has to admit that there is something not quite perfect about her. Something not quite right. So the search has to go on. But by now it's as though the more he searches, the more impossible it becomes to actually find her. He says he sometimes feels quite desperate. Trapped in this endless, circular quest, he has obviously not heard Franz Kafka's remark that 'the Messiah will come only when he's no longer necessary; he will come only on the day after his arrival'.

For a moment I come awake. There is something I have to ask of him, but it's difficult to interrupt the rapid flow of his words, rushing like a speeding express train towards me. But what would happen, I ask eventually, when he pauses for breath, if she were ever to arrive? How would he feel if he were actually to meet her. In the flesh, as it were. If one day there was that sudden *coup de foudre*, that instant recognition? And his parents agreed. What would happen next? For a moment he looks vague and uncertain. He pours some more of the cold tea into his cup, but none into mine. I can see him asking himself that question, as if for the first time. Then he smiles; a beatific look settles on his plump face. He voice seems flat, and rehearsed. He talks as if that moment would somehow usher in the end of his personal History, and the beginning of an entirely new era. A time of freedom from all anxieties and struggle, a state of pure, but ill-defined, bliss. Meeting her, he says, would mean the total healing of all previous wounds and disappointments, the fulfilment of every dream. As if he would live from then on in a timeless, numinous world. A sort of private millennium.

Suddenly, without warning, he stands up and begins to gather his things together, collect his suitcase from the rack above him, fold up his newspaper, getting ready to leave at the next station. But the train has slowed down, and just before we arrive, he finishes the story, though he no longer seems aware of the listener sitting across from him. For the results of this lifetime myth have been both tragic and predictable – a long succession of failed relationships, and a cluster of angry ex-fiancées. But despite all of this, he says, standing over me, his face serious now, he hasn't lost hope. He will still continue to search for Her. He just cannot stop. Every moment he waits and waits anxiously for Her arrival. In the meantime, all his vague feelings of hope and anticipation seem to have crystallised into a type of faith, almost a private religion, though one with only a single devotee. It seems to me that after so many disappointments, this Myth of the Future is about all that he has to keep his growing despair at bay.

As the ancient Romans used to say, '*Spes ultima dea*' – Hope is the last Goddess. Or, in this case: Godette.

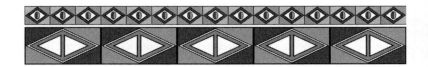

CHAPTER
7

HEALING AND CURING

*'Writing prescriptions is easy, but coming to an understanding with
people is hard.'*

Franz Kafka, 'A Country Doctor'

Mr H is a grey, elderly, stooped man. He always wears the same
flat cloth cap, the same patched grey jacket and crumpled
shirt, whenever he comes to see me at the Medical Centre. He
has the accent and manner of a countryman, but one now marooned in
the big city, living with his married daughter for many years, ever since
his wife died. He is a practical man, with strong hands and broken fingernails, and a darkly tanned skin speckled with liver spots, A man of
silences, or of very few words, humble and awkward. He never meets my
eye. I get to know him only slightly over weeks, then over months, while
I am working as a locum doctor in that area. He is always monosyllabic,
withdrawn, perhaps depressed. I know nothing about him, or about his
past.

One day, after I have measured his blood pressure and given him
the usual one-month prescription for his tablets, he unexpectedly
leans forward. Silently, he takes something out of a big plastic bag that
he's brought with him, and carefully places it on my desk. It is a flat
rectangular object, wrapped in thick brown paper, and tied with old
thick string. For a moment I think he has brought me a present. His
face is fixed in concentration as he slowly folds back the layers of paper,

to reveal his treasure. It is a long black-and-white photograph, carefully framed. It shows the deck of a Royal Navy battleship, sometime before or during the Second World War. It seems to have been taken in port after a tour of duty at sea, or perhaps just before. In Portsmouth, I think he said. The photograph is formal, and carefully arranged. It shows hundreds of the ship's company assembled on deck, in stiff, serried, uniformed rows. Right in the foreground, if you look carefully, is the tiny figure of King George VI in naval uniform, tall and serious, surrounded by the ship's senior officers.

Mr H points, with a gnarled, shaking, arthritic finger at a tiny pale face, in the second-last row on the right, surrounded by hundreds of other pale faces of young sailors. His face brightens. At that moment, time collapses. Decades disappear. He is a young man again, that young Ordinary Seaman, not the old man with the ruined, disappointed face and the wasted body. To him that day seems to have been one of the key moments, maybe *the* moment, in a humble life – a point of intersection with famous personalities and great historical dramas. It's the first time I've ever seen him smile. His few remaining teeth are yellowed and irregular, and stained with tobacco.

'It's a picture of me, doctor,' he says with a shy pride. 'That's *me*, up here. And down here on the deck – *that is King George!*'

We sit in silence as I examine the photograph, holding it up close to my face. For just a moment I find myself back in Cape Town, sitting on my father's shoulders in Adderley Street as this same King, his Queen and two Princesses drive slowly past us and everyone waves flags and cheers. The year is 1947, and not so many years after the photograph was taken.

We share the moment. He is relaxed now, proud in his achievement, his moment in History. Maybe his blood pressure has even dropped a little. We talk more about that day, and what it meant to him. After a while he leaves, still smiling and carefully clutching his plastic bag. It's only a trivial incident, of course, but we have forged a sort of relationship now. Before my eyes he has metamorphosed from a patient into a person. It's a priceless moment, and I know that it will last. But you certainly won't find it described in any medical textbook.

It's much too trivial for that.

Several weeks later, and an old woman whom I hardly know suddenly opens her bag, rummages around, and then takes out to show me a photograph of her latest grandchild, living overseas. She talks and talks, but not about her diabetes or her blood pressure. She, too, leaves smiling, more relaxed than she was before. And then there is that other very old man – also colourless, silent, wary and withdrawn – who suddenly comes to life when I mention how much I like jazz, boasting to me of his extensive collection of old jazz LPs, and how as a lad during the Second World War he had actually heard the great Glenn Miller himself, and his big band, playing at a US airbase in East Anglia. He is proud to have been there that day, and proud of his vast knowledge of modern music. And proud, too, that he knows much more about jazz than I ever will.

I will never know why these small events happened, and at those particular times. They were never planned. But each one reminds me, forcefully, that in medicine there's no such thing as an ordinary patient. Simple or anonymous, each one has a story to tell, if only one has the time and the patience to listen. And sometimes that listening is every bit as important as testing their blood sugars, or examining their lungs.

These examples remind me that medicine is not just about disease. It's also about health – or rather, about the healthy parts of people's lives. And yet healthy, contented people, in harmony with their lives, are a rare sight in clinical practice, and their absence is a huge and significant void. It can become part of the *déformation professionnelle* of every doctor, a distorted world-view. And healthy people are completely absent, too, from all my medical textbooks. Paging through those plump, hard-backed volumes on my shelf, all I can see, on one glossy page after another, are photographs of wounded or infected bodies, of unhappy people broken by injury or disease. Sick and suffering people who come in to see me every day of the week, coughing, sighing, or grimacing with pain.

But contrary to those books, experience teaches me that, in a sense, *everyone* is healthy – even if they are dying. For even then, there's always some small undamaged bit that remains behind: an ironic joke, a sudden flicker of hope, a comment on politics, or some tiny morsel of gossip. Something from the deep past, maybe, like the pride of a young sailor on the deck of a wartime battleship, many decades ago. Focusing on that small area of wellness can help to create, if for only an instant, a very different atmosphere. It can take a person away into an alternative reality, but one that is just as real. Far away from the thick, foetid atmosphere of the sickroom, or the hospital ward, with their odours of despair, and the sense of time compressed, so that to them minutes come to seem like hours, and hours elongate into days.

I think of another old man lying alone in his house. How the air inside his room feels thick, condensed, the voices of his nurses and doctors shrill and wavering, as if all of us had been inhaling helium. The old man is alone, and lonely, and waiting for the end. I know that it won't be long now. I see the bowl at the bedside with its blood-stained phlegm and, under the bed like a carafe of white wine, a plastic bottle half-filled with urine. It is a room of low voices and forced smiles, of long looks and gentle nudges.

I sit myself down at his bedside, my black medical bag resting on my lap. The small table beside me is crowded with glass bottles and plastic containers of pills, powders and mixtures, with bottles of mineral water and cartons of high protein drinks and dietary supplements. Next to them lies a random assemblage of rubber tubes and swabs, strips of gauze and little transparent sachets of saline, as well as piles of disposable syringes – each in its own, private, plastic packet. A tall grey oxygen cylinder stands in one corner of the room, attached to the man's nostrils by a thin, blue plastic tube. Stuck to the wall with sticking tape, just above his head, is a rota of his carers, for night and for day. A faint, antiseptic smell rises from the wheeled commode, parked in a distant corner of the room. Time has congealed in that room, and hope too.

And yet here we are, quite unexpectedly, arguing politics. Mr M was active in the trade union movement as a young man, so many years ago. He still has strong opinions about this government policy or that, and despite his terminal illness he seems to be quite up to date with the latest news, the latest strikes or government policies, the most recent developments in industrial relations. For a moment, Mr M comes back to life. He raises himself on his thin elbows, becomes angry, even a little flushed. He wags his thin, skeletal fingers at me. In his frail, wavering voice he attacks one government minister after another, scorns a particular politician recently in the news, praises another, speaks dismissively of the popular press, sneers at some fellow trade-unionists for their recent no-strike agreements with their employers in Big Business. For a moment the young firebrand re-emerges in that room of death, full of his old rage and sharp opinions, his hopes and dreams for a better world. The fatal ticking of the clock, and the smells of dying, all disappear. But then suddenly Mr M becomes exhausted again, and falls back into the stained pillows with a sigh. The whole incident has only lasted a moment, and yet for that brief instant we have escaped from that room – travelled to somewhere else, a place far away from death. He's had a tiny holiday in a healthier place.

He coughs deeply into the bowl again, splutters, retches, sinks into bed again, his face putty-coloured now and covered with sweat. Then he looks up and notices that I am still standing at his bedside.

'That bloody prime minister,' he begins again, 'it's all *her* fault… .'

Dr L is an old family doctor, battle-weary and cynical after decades in practice. He's a traditional, no-nonsense type of doctor, stern and im-patient, though he has a warm and kindly core. He's full of advice to me about the tiny things, the ones that really make a difference to patient care, but are never mentioned in my medical textbooks.

'Whenever you see those old, lonely people,' he says (and here he doesn't include himself), 'all those widows, and those sad old widowers, always make sure that you *touch* them, even very lightly, during the consultation. Shake their hands, tap them on the shoulder, maybe even put your arm around them.' In a country like this, he explains, so emotionally distant, so non-tactile, many of these old folks are hardly ever touched. Month after month, nobody ever hugs them, or cuddles them, or strokes their withered faces. No-one reminds them that they still exist. 'Some of them hardly ever see their families, you know, even though they live nearby.'

'It's really sad,' he adds, putting his hand for a moment on my shoulder, and then shaking his head. 'It's pitiful, really. I can't change this country, but – well, it's the least that I can do… .'

For all his authoritarian air, Dr L is humorous and warm. He tickles the children, jokes with their parents, flirts with the old ladies ('What do you mean, you're 73. *That's not old!* I've got a nice young man to introduce you to – and he's only 76!'), talks football, investments or war experiences with each of the older men.

One after another the old folks leave his room, smiling, glowing, contented. Some even giggling. For Dr L has reminded them that they are people who just happen to have a disease – and not the other way round. They're more than a diagnosis dressed up in a suit or a dress. He makes them feel seen, listened to, alive. Over the decades he has healed very many of them, even if he hasn't always been able to cure their physical ills. Every time I see him at work, he reminds me that medical practice is about all those tiny, trivial, almost invisible things. They're the ones that really make a difference. And Dr L is full of advice about them.

'And don't ever forget about *time*, he says. 'Always pay attention to time – and the ways that it can affect your patients' bodies and their minds.' He warns me that time is never linear; and that in emotional terms it can loop and curve back on itself, at any particular moment. And that some traumatic memories can act like time-bombs, set to go off at some unexpected time in the future.

His words come back sharply to me in the summer of 1994. That is the year of the 50th anniversary celebrations of the Normandy D-Day landings, and there is saturation coverage of that momentous event in newspapers and magazines, and on every television screen. A number of old soldiers, who had taken part in the landings, suddenly sink without warning into deep depressions. They develop nightmares and fearful flashbacks. Up till that moment they had been strong, phlegmatic, unemotional men. They had coped well with their lives, and tried never to look back at the War. Now the War has caught up with them again, and they are no longer allowed their amnesia. Every day their own memories of those terrible times stare back at them from newspapers, or from the TV screen.

One year later, in 1995, and all of this repeats itself. This time it is another group of elderly people who sit across the desk from me – men or women with pale, haunted faces, some with blue numbers still tattooed on their arms. They, too, have developed nightmares and depression and horrific flashbacks. It is now the 50th anniversary of the liberation of the Nazi concentration camps – Belsen, Dachau, Auschwitz, Ravensbruck and the rest – in the last year of the War. Once again the television screens are full of those awful, grainy newsreels of piles of naked corpses, of broken people in striped rags wandering like ghosts among the soldiers who had just liberated them. These elderly people have also coped well until then, and also got on with their lives. But now it has all come back to haunt them; it is as if the past had reached forward in time, and with its cold skeletal hand, gripped them tightly again.

Someone at the time called it the '50-Year Syndrome', and it broke the spirits of some of those survivors. Like the 'anniversary reactions' of depression so common on the exact date of a past bereavement, it shows the power of the calendar over the human body, and mind. Like the surge in stress symptoms among accountants at the end of the tax year, or in students at their end-of-year exams, many people are victims of time – of the tyranny of the calendar, the clock, the timetable, as well as of rigid schedules and appointment times.

'Just think about all the effects on their bodies,' says Dr L, shaking his head. 'Of all those awful "rush hours" that they have to endure, twice a day, five days a week, on trains and buses and cars. What does that do to their nerves, as well as their coronary arteries? Think of that middle-aged man in the business suit sitting over there in the waiting room, glancing frantically down at his watch, his heart pump-pump-pumping away in his chest, his bloodstream full of high-octane adrenaline, his body in constant conflict with that watch on his wrist. Think of him. Poor sod. He's not the master of his life. He's the slave. So if you want to help him, and prevent that heart attack, look beyond him, at all that pressure that time puts upon him. Try to free him from his addiction to time. That's the trick. Get him to release himself from that particular slavery – instead of just treating his raised blood pressure.'

Dr L's advice is the very opposite of that offered by Benjamin Franklin in 1736, in a canny essay called *Necessary Hints to Those That Would Be Rich*. Even in those days, Dr Franklin saw how intertwined time was with money, but he was completely unaware of the consequences to health of this entanglement. 'He that idly loses five shillings worth of time,' he wrote, 'loses five shillings, and might as prudently throw five shillings into the sea. He that loses five shillings, not only loses that sum, but all the advantages that might be made by turning it in dealing, which by the time that a young man becomes old, will amount to a considerable sum of money.'

'So that's why you should always pay attention to time,' says Dr L, when I read him that quote. 'For that sort of pressure can easily destroy a man, wreck his marriage, and damage his heart.'

Then he looks down suddenly at his wristwatch. 'Got to go,' he says, 'Sorry. Got to rush. I've got a patient booked in at three.'

I admire old-style family doctors like Dr L, just as I admire many of the traditional healers or shamans that I've met through my anthropology studies, and for very similar reasons. Both are healers of the person, as well as curers of the body. And I admire their insight that 'health' is not just the absence of physical disease, but has many different dimensions to it, including the state of mind and of spirit, and the quality of relationships with other people.

But despite Dr L's advice, mainstream medicine – especially in those big, busy, urban hospitals – still concentrates primarily on the body, and on its many dysfunctions. However, most doctors soon realise that this approach doesn't work, for it can leave their patients feeling dissatisfied, bereft, and sometimes very angry.

Including Dr L, I have met six great doctors in my life – one of them my late uncle, a prominent gastroenterologist in Cape Town. Each of these men, or women, in their own way, was a great healer as well as an eminent medical scientist. Each had that same, quiet quality about them when they dealt with patients. Call it love, if you will, or a type of focused compassion. It was the way they became so silent and alert, how they seemed to use every sense that they possessed – sight, hearing, smell, touch, plus memory and intuition – to fully understand their patient's situation.

Once in a hospital ward, I stood watching one of them closely as he sat at the bedside of an elderly woman, holding her hand and nodding quietly whenever she spoke. I marvelled at how alert he was to her every nuance of expression, every tiny movement, whether quick or slow. The slow, careful questions he asked, and how receptive he was to her replies. For at that moment he seemed to have become an empty vessel, ready to be filled entirely by her story of suffering. At times when the diagnosis was unclear, he became like a hunter, whose prey was hidden within a jungle of confusing symptoms. He would stalk it patiently, taking his time. There was no hurry in his manner, no impatience or irritation, only a deep and penetrating silence, with an occasional murmured question.

And I noticed, too, that these cautious questions also dealt with the patient herself – her family and her feelings, and how she viewed her condition. Only when he'd got the whole picture in his grasp, would he begin her treatment. To heal her, as well as to cure her.

At times medical practice reminds me of a certain type of archaeology. For the reality is that most patients present their doctors with only the broken shards of a human life – the one's labelled infection, disease, suffering and pain. But each of these shards is only a small part of a much larger picture. And in order to understand it fully, the doctor will have to try and reconstruct the rest. Above all, to try to imagine all those other healthy, ordinary, aspects of their lives that patients leave behind whenever they enter his room. Their work and love lives, their homes, their marriages and children, the hidden world of their hobbies, and the rich stores of memories that each one carries around. And then, like one of those rebuilt Greek vases in the British Museum – where only a few of the original shards still exist – to try to see that person's life as a whole again – as it must have looked before it was shattered, and the fragments all dispersed. A life that, despite its missing bits and mended cracks, was once a unity, a coherent and functional thing.

That's why fine doctors like Dr L always tell us to learn as much as possible about our patients, and who they are outside their patient role. Those aspects that can sometimes be glimpsed from afar, smiling and chatting in the pub or the supermarket, or staring back at you proudly from a wartime photograph. And then try and work with those healthy parts for the patient's recovery, and not regard them either an irrelevance or an enemy. For especially in chronic diseases, medical treatment is a joint project. After all, who will care for the patient when the doctor is not around? Who will choose to take enough exercise or eat a proper diet, or give up smoking, or regularly take their medication or insulin injections? It's a way of giving the patient back some control over his, or her. disease, and in the process, probably enhancing his general health, as well as his resistance to disease.

The textbooks offer me no specific advice on how to do this. They are always made up of standard types, generalisations, composites, a parade of 'typical cases' paraded through page after page. They are rarely about individuals, except when those individuals are used to illustrate a particular example of a disease. And that's how it should be. It's the most efficient way of transmitting knowledge to medical students. But this one-size-fits-all approach is also limited. And only experience can teach that lesson.

But a certain mystery still remains. Why are some doctors able to heal their patients' minds, and repair their lives – while others simply cannot? After all, both groups have had very similar medical training. And why can I myself sometimes cure someone, but then fail to heal them? I still don't fully understand. Dr L has given me some clues, but the real answer still remains elusive.

But whatever it is, it means that medicine can never be purely a science. It is too human an activity for that. It is also a literary art, for it is as much about creativity and imagination, and the stories that patients tell, or don't tell, as about their blood tests or electrocardiograms. To truly heal as well as cure requires the doctor to empathise, but also to *imagine* what it must be like to be that particular person sitting across the desk from you, looking up at you anxiously from the hospital bed, or being wheeled swiftly past into the operating theatre. It requires an act of the imagination, as well as of the heart.

Yet for all his folksy wisdom, old Dr L is surprisingly up to date on the latest medical research, the latest modes of treatment. Each week he reads the medical journals, as soon as they arrive. He carries piles of them around on the back seat of his ancient car. He illustrates that the scientific approach, and technology, of medicine is vital to health care, and is quite irreplaceable.

But as he always reminds me, 'Science is necessary. You know that. But at the same time it is never, ever sufficient.'

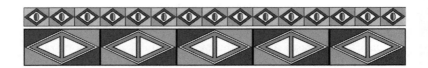

CHAPTER 8

THE PSYCHE AND THE SOMA

'The sorrow which has no vent in tears, may make other organs weep.'

Dr Henry Maudsley, 1918

Yes, but what does that word *mean*?' I ask her again. 'What do *you* think the doctors mean when they tell you that your condition is partially "psychosomatic"? What do they actually mean by that word?'

It's in the mid-1980s. I am in the USA carrying out a research project at one of the teaching hospitals of Harvard Medical School. It's a study of how people perceive psychosomatic disorders – conditions that are not only physical, but which also have some strong emotional component, or in some cases, a psychological cause. I'm particularly interested in those who suffer from certain abdominal conditions, such as nervous vomiting, the irritable bowel syndrome (IBS) and ulcerative colitis. All the people that I interview have been told by their physicians, over many years, that their illnesses have a strong 'psychosomatic' component. But what do they mean by that word?

I meet them one by one in a small waiting room on the ground floor, with the hospital tannoy system booming in the background. We sit on sagging chairs on either side of a small formica table covered with coffee stains, while I make notes and transcribe their words.

The woman I'll call Diane is in her mid-30s, with a round worried face, rimless spectacles, and a distant, distracted air. At first she finds it difficult to understand my accent, but then slowly she relaxes and begins to talk. She says her ulcerative colitis causes frequent attacks of bloody diarrhoea and abdominal pains, often without warning. She's had the condition for many years now and so far medical treatment hasn't helped her much, nor prevented these unwelcome attacks. Her doctor has suggested to her that I should interview her, as part of my study.

'What do you think caused your illness?' I ask.

She answers my question slowly, deliberately, but there's a deep anger in her voice.

'They tell me it's a lot of genetic tendencies to put psychological stress into my body,' she says. 'Until a year ago the doctors were telling me I was crazy. It was my own fault because of what I did. Some said it's because of how you ate. Some said because I was too sensitive. Others said it was because of exercise. Others said because I wasn't taking enough Azulfidine. What I hear from all the doctors was that it was my fault, and if only you did what they said, everything would be OK. Catherine, my doctor, she asked me what "psychosomatic" meant. She said, "It's not what you think – people think that psychosomatic means that it's your fault" – but she says that there's a genetic tendency to put stress in your body, and that's a weakness you have. Before Catherine, they said it was all my fault, and that if only I did things differently everything would be OK.'

'Why does the disease affect that particular part of your body?' I ask.

Diane takes a deep breath. 'Doctors often say anger gets stored in the colon,' she explains, 'and someone who's read my chart says my colon's weak. Stress goes to the weakest organ, you know. I let it get to me, and eat me away. Once something gets inside of me it just bounces around inside of me, until I can get rid of it. If I can catch anger while it's fresh and pound something, I'll get it out of me – or someone will help me get it out.'

Diane blames herself for her condition. She says it comes from being much too sensitive, from caring much too deeply. 'Worry weakens the body,' she says, 'and the constant worry puts stress on the weakened organ of the body, which in my case was the colon.'

Annie, the next woman I interview, also blames herself. 'People who have a short fuse are unlikely to be affected by it,' she says. 'You would just blow up and get all the anger out. Someone who tears himself apart [gets it]. It's not expressing anger, bottling anger up.'

A young man named Brett tells me how many people that he knows, including his doctors, are blaming him unfairly for his colitis. 'Other people were all saying that there was something wrong with me psychologically,' he says, shaking his head. '[But] if I'd had appendicitis or a cough, I would have been spared this. Some of these friends were doctors, others not. They say it's often associated with a psychological component. I searched very hard and for a reason. Why *me*? Everyone told me it *must* be psychological,' he says. 'There *must* be a large psychological component – it's in the medical textbooks. Our society associates the bowel and stomach with nervousness – it's more sensitive to tension.'

The following week I interview three women, each suffering from the unpredictable diarrhoea, cramps and flatulence of IBS. All have their own theories about why they get ill. 'I tend to hold lots of things inside,' says one 34-year-old. 'I don't express emotion freely. Anger, tension, hostility, fear; any kind of upset – I think of them as being crammed into my colon.' '[It's] probably because I don't get wrinkles, and I don't get heart attacks,' says a 27-year-old, 'and the tension has to go somewhere – so it went to my bowel… Probably some people hold tension in the stomach, and others hold it further up, and I've heard that you hold anger in your stomach, and sadness in your jaw.' A woman of 30 has a similar idea. She gets attacks of diarrhoea whenever she's upset. It comes, she says, from 'maybe not letting anger out. Even today if I'm angry with someone, I can get an attack. But I can't let my anger out… When you're angry and you can't let it out, it causes tension, and that's connected to your nerves, and it's a way of releasing itself – instead of angry words, it come out like this.' 'You have to find a way of letting it out,' she adds. 'If you hold it in it can make you sick.' 'You get sick if you don't unload a lot of anger,' adds another woman, with nervous vomiting.

I have never before heard anger described in this way, nor this hydraulic model of the blockage and flow of emotions. It's almost as if anger itself were a toxic, purulent liquid. As though, if it were to accumulate inside a person, and not be released very soon, it could turn dangerous – become a festering abscess, filled with pus.

The study progresses, week after week. But one word, recurring in most of the interviews, increasingly puzzles me. What is this 'It' that Diane and the others constantly refer to? What is this mysterious, malevolent entity – the one they also call '*stress*', or sometimes 'tension'? This vague and invisible force that somehow 'enters' their bodies, mutates into anger, and then causes them to vomit, run to the toilet or have stomach cramps? Especially as this evil entity is apparently capable of transforming itself from the invisible to the visible, from the intangible to the material – and then back again. Appearing either as an emotion or words, or as something purely physical like faeces or vomit.

The more I hear about 'It', the more it seems that, half-hidden in their words, is the spoor of a much older idea. And the more it reminds me of something I've read long before – in one of my anthropology books at university. It was in the chapter on 'spirit possession', the one all about those malevolent spirits said to 'possess' people in more traditional societies. Like 'It', these people also describe an invisible force that originates outside of their body, and which then 'enters' them. It's something out there, in the air, invisible, inherent in certain relationships, or in some types of work situation. Once this toxic entity has entered your body, it can make you ill or unhappy, or even drive you insane. It can only be expelled by a ritual of exorcism.

Or – in a modern society like ours – by another type of ritual: expressing it, talking it through, sharing it with other people, and with their help 'getting it off your chest'.

'You won't get ill,' says a woman with nervous vomiting to me, 'if you have people you can confide in, can unload on, so that you're not carrying emotional stress along.' 'You get sick if you don't unload a lot of anger,' says another. 'A good relationship can make you stay healthy, because you can ventilate a lot of stress,' adds a third.

It appears that in order to wreak most damage, this 'It' needs an ally. Like Diane's colon, it needs a weak, unreliable organ within the body on which to act, a body part that is especially vulnerable. A gap in one's defences. A traitor within.

Once 'It' has entered the body, it heads straight for that 'weak organ'.

A woman with IBS takes a deep breath, shrugs. 'If there's a basic weakness in the body [it goes there],' she says, 'that's why it affects that part of the body. That's the weakest part for it to go.' Another, with ulcerative colitis, points down at her lower tummy. 'I feel I *do* have a target organ,' she says, frowning. 'If something goes wrong, the old colon gets it.'

They speak of these organs as if they were, in some way, autonomous. As if they were also a type of 'It', with their own independent existence, even their own volition. They are foreigners, resident aliens within the body, and only partly under their control. They have to be monitored continuously, and on occasion even negotiated with. As a woman with IBS puts it, she can control her symptoms only by 'trying to monitor what's happening. Being in touch with what's inside before the colon knows. Using relaxation. Talking to the various organs. It helps.'

In 1976 a New York physician, Eric J Cassell, described how his patients often spoke of their diseases, or a diseased organ, as an 'it' – as an object apart from themselves. In ways similar to my own study, it was as if these were 'independent entities', somehow independent of the person, and not under their full control. 'Now tell *it* to go away,' says a woman with breast cancer to him, pointing at the lump in her breast. Diseased organs were spoken of as '*the* breast', '*the* ovary', or '*the* eyes' – rather than '*my* breast', '*my* ovary', '*my* eyes'. He speculated that referring to malfunctioning body parts as if they were 'depersonalized objects' was a form of denial. It was the patients' way of protecting themselves, distancing themselves from the implications of their disease by somehow separating it off. It was almost as if that diseased organ belonged elsewhere – not in that particular body.

Cassell traced this view to a much older debate within medicine, from Hippocrates onwards. It was between the 'physiologists' – who believed that disease was the result of an imbalance within the human body, or between it and its environment – and the 'ontologists' – who believed that disease was 'an object or thing that invaded the body'. About 200 years ago this latter view became the dominant one, and the eventual rise of Germ Theory a century later sealed its victory. From then on, most diseases were seen as independent entities, often caused by the entry of other entities – such as 'germs' – into the body. Traces of the ontologists' theory of invasion can be found also in the early works of Sigmund Freud, as they are in the words of Diane and the others.

The historian K Codell Carter has described how much of Freud's early imagery from 1893 onwards was heavily influenced by the Germ Theory emerging at that time. Before then, diseases were identified not by a specific cause, but by a cluster of symptoms and observable changes in the body. In many medical tracts, causes were simply not mentioned. But once Koch had identified the TB bacillus in 1882, and Klebs had discovered the Diphtheria bacillus in 1884, medicine began to focus more on the specific *causes* of infections, and only then on their specific results. The names of diseases were gradually changed from sets of symptoms to the type of infection caused by a particular micro-organism.

'Freud's work on psychopathology,' wrote Carter, 'ended up exactly in harmony with the main orientation of the medical research of his time.' For the first time, Freud gave a coherent scientific explanation of nervous diseases. Before him, mental conditions such as 'hysteria' had been seen mainly as clusters of symptoms, and the causes given for them were vague and inconsistent. But like other medical scientists at that time, Freud started with the causes of these disorders – especially in a person's early sexual development – and then went on to the symptoms that resulted from them.

In their 1893 work, *On the Psychical Mechanism of Hysterical Phenomena*, Freud and Breuer had spoken of how 'psychical trauma' acts 'like a foreign body which long after its entry must continue to be regarded as an agent that is still at work'. They described how 'the treatment, too, worked like the removal of a foreign body from the living tissue.'

'I have described my treatment as psychotherapeutic operations,' Freud wrote, 'and I have brought out their analogy with the opening up of a cavity filled with pus, the scraping out of a carous region, etc.' He justified this abscess analogy not only 'by the removal of what is pathological', but also by 'the establishment of conditions that are more likely to lead the course of the process in the direction of recovery'.

To the people in my study, however, these ideas are not seen as analogies; they seem to be taken quite literally. They appear to be real to them, almost concrete. And what's more, their imagery is not that far from the spatial metaphors still commonly used in modern psychology, where the psyche is sometimes described as if it were a sort of 'box' with invisible walls that can be breached from within, or penetrated from without. In psychotherapy, wild emotions and thoughts need to be 'contained'; personal 'boundaries' need to be established; 'projections' and 'introjections' need to be recognised, and then analysed; bad feelings or memories 'repressed' too deeply, need to be revealed, and then got rid of – because if left in place they could become toxic waste products, and cause problems. In therapy, clients are often encouraged to get rid of bad feelings by catharsis – by 'expressing' them, 'talking it through', 'letting it all come out', or by 'getting it off their chests and not bottling it up'.

The theme of the 'invasion' of personal boundaries, and its subsequent cure by expulsion, dates not only from Freud, but from much earlier. And it is still here, right here in this small interview room, among this group of people who each carry around with them, like a heavy and painful burden, the diagnosis of 'psychosomatic'.

The actual word 'psychosomatic' has been around a long time (it was coined in 1818 by a German psychiatrist, Dr Heinroth), but it's only since World War Two that it's become so widely used. It was a revolutionary concept in its time, a sincere attempt to overcome the mind-body dualism inherent in Western medicine since the time of Descartes. It aimed to offer a holistic understanding of all the dimensions of illness, by unifying the phenomena of mind ('psyche') with those of the body ('soma').

Despite this noble aim, many of the early psychosomatic theories were tinged with strong moral disapproval. Some doctors suggested that each disorder was associated with a specific, abnormal 'personality type', 'personality trait' or 'character disturbance' – and which then contributed to its development. One, for example, described the so-called 'character structure' of ulcerative colitis patients as: 'They are fearful and when in imminent danger often overtly cowardly.' Others spoke of the 'consistent characterological features' of people with asthma, including 'unusually strong passive and dependent personality traits', and the need to get emotional support from people around them.

In 1968, a Dr Edwin Gildea tried to link certain specific traits, such as 'abnormal assertiveness' ('Rarely able to verbalise feelings even when aware of them. Just takes it from boss, wife, friends, etc'), to specific disorders, such as high blood pressure, peptic ulcers and rheumatoid arthritis. As late as the 1980s, two other researchers – Drs Cheren and Knapp – were describing the 'typical personality traits' or 'character disturbances' of patients suffering from Crohn's disease, as 'compulsive or paranoid traits' with excessive dependency, compliance and 'explosive manipulation'.

These days, almost all of these 'personality' theories, with their harsh judgemental tone, have been rejected by physicians. Solely blaming the patient's personality, or their behaviour, has largely gone out of fashion. As Catherine, Diane's doctor, had said to her, they've been challenged by more recent developments in medicine, especially in genetics and immunology, as well as by new approaches in psychology. But in the self-blame of Diane and the others, one can still detect the trace of those much older theories. Personality theories may have disappeared from most medical textbooks, but they haven't vanished from some of those who suffer from psychosomatic disorders – and nor has the idea of the invasion by 'It'.

As they tell it, it's been a particularly painful experience for them. The stigma, the shame, the embarrassment they feel, the way people like them are labelled 'psychosomatic', and often attract blame from others. The way some people even see these conditions as not quite real, as being largely imaginary and 'all in the mind'. As for their doctors, many of their patients think that some of them, too, blame them for getting ill in the first place – or else for failing to get better. The doctors seem to dislike this kind of illness because, unlike other conditions, it is often so difficult to predict or to control. These conditions tend to recur at unexpected times. They don't always respond to treatment. And they often make doctors feel helpless, frustrated, and sometimes very angry.

The people I meet through my study all live in a society that values youth, health, beauty and independence above all else, as well as full control over all bodily functions. It seems that in this milieu, some of those with psychosomatic disorders deal with the disapproval of others by shifting responsibility for the disorder away from themselves. They place it instead on those parts of their bodies that are 'weak', unreliable – parts for which they don't feel completely responsible, and over which they don't feel they have full control. It's a way of protecting their self-image, of keeping intact an idealised sense of self – one that conforms to society's expectations – by disowning those parts that don't quite fit. It means putting the blame onto 'nervous stomachs', 'irritable colons' or 'weak chests' – rather than onto their own nervousness, irritability or weakness.

But the price of conforming to this social ideal seems high. It means being left with only a shrunken Self inside. A tiny, youthful, perfectly healthy homunculus deep within, surrounded on all sides by 'weak' organs, dangerous emotions, or unreliable personality traits. A minute victim-Self under constant threat of attack from 'It' outside, or from a weakness within.

This is the story that Diane and the others seem to have learned. A story that carries with it a sharp, moralistic message.

'It's *your* neurotic or over-anxious personality that's the true culprit,' it says. '*That's* the cause of your condition; not anything about your body or its genetic make-up. Nor has it anything to do with the circumstances of your life, the pressures you are under, or the environment in which you live, love, or work – it's due to *you*. No-one else. Stress may come from outside, but – ultimately – *you* are the one who let it in.

'It's your psyche that's to blame. Not your soma.'

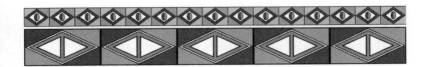

CHAPTER 9

DOUBLE DEATHS

Mid-morning, and as usual the old people have been seated in the 'solarium' of the Old Age Home. It's a large glass room on the top floor of the building, and the air within it is hot and stuffy, the big windows sealed, the central heating set much too high. There are the intermingled smells of floor polish, soap, disinfectant and the gradual decaying of aged bodies. Except for an occasional low murmur, the slow painful shuffle of a Zimmer frame, or the careful tap-tap of a walking stick along the faded carpets, the room is almost silent. There is almost no movement. You might think that everyone here was fast asleep. Somewhere in the background there is the faint electronic crackle of a television set, but its screen is out of focus: a flashing kaleidoscope of pictures like a constant visual hallucination. The sound level is set far too low to be heard, but too high to be completely ignored.

In their pink or blue dressing gowns and nightdresses, their pale smocks or faded pyjamas, the residents of the Home are sitting around the edge of the room. Some are slumped in their chairs; many seem to be heavily medicated. They remind me of a row of soft pastel plants arranged around an enormous greenhouse. Potted in their squashed slippers and swollen ankles, their stalks blue with varicose veins, each is topped with swaying fronds of thin, wispy, white hair, or sometimes with a bald head speckled with liver spots, Here and there, among the old ladies, I notice a faint line of mascara, a smear of lipstick around a toothless mouth, an irregular blush of rouge dabbed on by a shaking hand.

Three times a day in the greenhouse, the old people are fed and watered by the staff, but are otherwise ignored. Occasionally, though, you can hear the harsh, insistent tone of one of the carers, breaking the silence: '*That's* a good girl, Gladys! *Good girl!* Now take your other tablet.'

Many of these old folks, I've been told, have been completely abandoned by their families, others only partially so. On rare weekends when their daughters do come and visit (sometimes accompanied by an awkward son, or a bored grandchild), it must seem to them like *El Día de los Muertos*, the Day of the Dead. For this is a cemetery, only occupied by the living dead.

From time to time, but just for a moment, one of the corpses comes briefly to life. There is a sudden flurry of movement, or a few muttered words. Then silence again.

Despite these few, remaining sparks of the human spirit, I hate this place. I hate coming here, even when I have to do so to visit my own patients. It often makes me angry. It always fills me with despair.

Driving away, I am thinking how that big building is more than just an ante-chamber to death. In a way it is death itself, or a version of it. For it is filled with people trapped in a limbo-land, awkwardly suspended between one reality and another, between this world and the next. They are the undead, the unburied – shadowy spectres to be feared, avoided and shunned.

Their plight echoes a phenomenon that the anthropologist Roger Hertz once wrote about, and which he called the 'double death'. For he described how, in all human societies, people always die twice. First there's the death of their physical body – and then, after a period of time, this is followed by their 'social death'. This is the end of their personal identity, the one to which society says farewell at their funeral. Death is a long process, wrote Hertz, rather than a single point in time. It is a slow goodbye that can take many years, or even decades, to complete. It is the slow ending of a social identity, but also the beginning of a new one – as an ancestor, a forebear, a spirit, a fading photograph on the wall. But in the Old Age Home, this universal sequence of deaths seems to have been reversed. Despite all their grey-haired wisdom, their rich stores of memory and experience, the old people have not only been abandoned by society and their families. They have been declared dead, even though they are still alive.

I had seen this situation already long before, in my childhood in South Africa, when I used to visit my father at the state mental hospitals where he worked as a senior state psychiatrist. It was the way that the human life-span seemed to have become speeded up, condensed. The patients forcefully projected forward in time in order to transform themselves, without any delay, into their own ghosts: wrinkled, pale, insubstantial things, shambling along the corridors in their anonymous pyjamas, or frozen in silent tableaux on the stairway. Spectral figures, almost transparent to everyone around them.

Some weeks later I am standing in a small suburban house, occupied by a small suburban couple. The man has just been discharged home from the hospital after a diagnosis of cancer, but his treatment there has been proceeding favourably, and the hospital specialists are confident that his outlook is rather good. They expect him to live, for some years at least, if he looks after himself and continues to take his treatment. Now he lies in his bed with a pale, worried face, while I talk encouragingly about his situation. But he seems distracted, asking me question after question each time I try to leave the room, as if he really doesn't want me to leave him alone in there. Standing besides me, his wife is silent, withdrawn. She says hardly anything. But a few minutes later, on the landing outside his room, her demeanour suddenly changes. Her voice becomes brusque, her stare hard and cold. And yet there is something distracted about her, too, something distant and vague, as though like him she is only partly here, and already living elsewhere – in another time, another place. I give her precise instructions about his diet, his bodily care and other treatment, but she doesn't seem to be listening. Under her distant and empty stare, I can feel my optimistic voice beginning to falter and fade away. Suddenly she blurts out, 'How long will it be, doctor? I need to know *now*. I need to make the funeral arrangements.'

There is silence, except for the muffled ticking of clocks in different rooms, the deep coughing from the bedroom behind us, the rapid sounds of my own heartbeat. I am shocked. I try quickly to reassure her that his death is certainly *not* imminent. I babble on about 'reasonable prognosis' and 'good life expectancy for his age', and all the rest, but she seems to ignore me. She's not listening again.

'Look, doctor, ' she says, interrupting me. 'Look, I've been through this once already. With my first husband. He also died of cancer, you know. I went through hell that time, and I'm damn well *not* going through all that again. Not for anything.'

I carry on trying to be upbeat, but she seems implacable. And then a few weeks later, or maybe months, the man dies. The autopsy shows that, physically at least, it was a natural death due to his condition, and that there were no suspicious circumstances. But its timing is completely unexpected. It had happened much earlier than I and the other doctors anticipated.

Gradually I come to understand that when I visited him at his home, the man was already dead. After I left, his wife had done the necessary tasks, given him the necessary food and tablets, but that was all. She had withdrawn all love and hope and care from him. She had turned him into a living corpse. It was her way, I suppose, of protecting herself from the pain, and from the re-awakening of an earlier pain. Like the elderly people in the Old Age Home, her husband had already been declared dead. After that, the death of his body was almost an afterthought. An irrelevance.

Medical practice illustrates daily the enormous power of words, and the destructive power of a diagnostic label. The careless use of powerful words like 'cancer', 'heart attack', 'AIDS', or even 'mental illness', can sometimes damage and destroy. Especially when the diagnosis is given without offering any hope or comfort at the same time; without a plan of treatment or palliation, and with little awareness of the patient's feelings. In these situations, words can break the patient's morale, and rob him, or her, of hope. They can damage both body and mind. They can also lead other people to shun the patient, make excuses not to visit – just at the time when he needs them most. For some they provoke a fear of contagion (even the contagion of 'bad luck'). For others it is the mirror of their own mortality that keeps them away.

When the results of her tests have finally come through, Lorraine is seen at the hospital by a new doctor. A young man, tall and smart in a pressed white coat, with tightly combed hair, a shiny name-tag and a neat row of pens in his breast pocket. She has never met him before. The young doctor shuffles through the papers on the desk before him, takes a deep breath and then, staring intently at her, begins to speak.

It appears that this doctor sees himself as a very modern sort of physician, one who 'shares' all the information that he has with his patients. Who keeps nothing back. He is certain that he's completely unlike all those old-fashioned doctors of previous generations, with their paternalism and carefully crafted mystique, their dependant and uninformed patients. He strongly believes in 'information' and 'facts', and in offering them freely to patients – but is less interested in the effect that these facts may have on them. That's not his problem, he feels. It's the patient's. After all, patients are rational, autonomous adult beings who deserve all the information available, and on that basis they can then make an informed choice about their lives.

'I'm not into any power trips,' he always says to his colleagues. 'I believe in total equality between doctor and patient – in an educated and informed patient population. I believe the patient should know *exactly* what I know.'

He looks up again from her medical file. 'Look, Lorraine,' he says, 'I'll be honest with you. And you're entitled to know. Your prognosis is poor. *Very* poor. According to the latest studies…' and here he gestures to a pile of medical journals stacked neatly on his desk, '67 per cent of people with your condition will die within the first six months. It is 67, isn't it? … Hold on, just let me check. Yes, that's the latest figure from the Mayo Clinic study. So that's it. I'm afraid you need to get your affairs in order. You really have my sympathy.'

He rises from his chair, smiles, firmly shakes her hand, and then ushers her – sobbing and gasping – out of the room. The question remains hovering in the air behind her – is he cruel or insensitive, or just very inexperienced? But Lorraine and her family have no time to find out the answer. They are too distraught. For every moment from then on she feels doomed, sentenced to an imminent death. She too, has become one of the living dead.

Because the moment they hear what the hospital doctor has said to her, some of her friends begin acting oddly. Except for the very closest ones, they begin to withdraw from her. They make excuses. They are busy, *very* busy, they say. When they do come and see her, their voices are shrill and unnatural, or they speak in low, solicitous tones. They have fixed smiles on their faces. They sigh a lot. She finds that no-one ever argues with her. Everyone seems to agree with her, no matter what she says. And they laugh noisily, awkwardly if ever she makes a joke. And when they leave her house – hugging her closely, their voices breaking – she always feels much worse than she did before.

In fact Lorraine lives in reasonably good health for very much longer, but the damage to her morale has already been done.

Lorraine, the old people in the Home, and the man in that small suburban house, are all examples of what the physician George Engel once called the 'given-up-giving-up complex'. It's a sense of profound hopelessness and futility, of abandonment by all those around you, of the future being suddenly snatched away. In his studies in the USA, Engel found that often this leads to illness in the victims, or even to sudden death. At its most extreme, it's a situation that anthropologists call 'voodoo death'.

They've reported it from many parts of the world – mainly from pre-industrial communities in parts of Africa, Australia, Latin America and the Caribbean. It's a form of social death that is created, and sustained, by the beliefs and expectations of that particular culture.

It happens usually in small rural communities when some powerful figure within the tribe – a sorcerer, religious leader or chief – publicly places a curse on a particular individual for breaking some religious taboo, or for committing a major crime. From that moment onwards, everyone around the victim regards him as doomed. His family, friends and all the community withdraw from him. They stop speaking to him, ignore him when he talks to them, stare straight through him as though he were not there. They see him as already dead, a walking corpse. He has become almost invisible to them, a shadowy vestige of his former self. He is there, but he is also not there.

The French anthropologist Claude Levi-Strauss has described what happens next. He writes how 'the victim yields to the combined terror, the sudden total withdrawal of the multiple reference systems provided by the support of the group, and, finally, to the group's decisive reversal in proclaiming him – once a living man, with rights and obligations – dead and an object of fear, ritual, and taboo.' In many such cases of voodoo death, people who believe they've been marked out in this way soon sicken and die. It usually happens within a few days, and apparently of natural causes.

In all its various forms, exotic or familiar, voodoo death illustrates that life is a fragile thing. It shows the power of words, and of words over flesh. How something intangible – like a curse or a medical diagnosis – can injure, and even kill. And it shows how we all need other people around to affirm that we're still alive; that we still exist as a person, and not just as a solid form of ghost, like one of the shadowy undead in the Old Age Home.

At first everyone thinks that Mrs P is depressed. She is a short, sprightly woman in her early 70s, a widow living alone in a small apartment. She has turned that apartment into a shrine of celebration to her late husband, her children and her growing brood of grandchildren. On the mantelpiece, the bookshelves, the chest of drawers, and the bedside table – among vases of flowers, miniature teapots, and rows of tiny porcelain statuettes – there is a crowded display of dozens of photographs. Weddings, engagements, graduations, babies gurgling or grimacing in cots, adolescents carrying prizes or footballs, and several sepia photographs in old silver frames of her own parents or grandparents, or of her wedding day.

And yet to her children Mrs P seems to be not quite herself. She is not concentrating too well, and is occasionally confused. And they notice, at times, that she's becoming quite forgetful. She forgets names and dates, even important birthdays and anniversaries, and often asks the same question repeatedly, again and again, like an old-fashioned gramophone needle caught in a groove. At times she has about her a distant, distracted air, as if she were there in the room, but also not there. At other times she seems more focused, just like her old self. Occasionally too she gets agitated and anxious, especially when she realises that she's forgotten some fact, or a name that she once knew well. Or – yet again – has left the lights on, or the gas fire burning when she last went out of her apartment. And yet she still seems to remember, often in amazing detail, some of the specific incidents of her youth, even of her early childhood. One of her daughters is convinced that she's really depressed, and that it's been developing gradually ever since her husband passed away from an unexpected heart attack almost two years before. Her sisters and brother are not so sure, but they all agree that something needs to be done. Something needs to be looked into. Eventually, at their urging, Mrs P agrees to go and see a doctor.

He examines her fully, but can find nothing wrong with her physically. Her heart function and lungs and blood pressure are all fine, and all the other tests are also normal, including those on her blood and urine. But he agrees that she does seem rather forgetful, even though he's noticed how emotionally flat she is, compared with before. He agrees that probably her 'cognitive loss' is a temporary one, and is really the indirect manifestation of her deep depression. It's quite common in her age group, he says, and as a therapeutic trial he will prescribe a course of anti-depressant tablets for her. The family bring her back to her apartment. In the next few weeks, everyone notices how she seems to have become more animated, less lethargic. She smiles a lot more, and at night sleeps a deeper sleep. And yet her memory does not improve. In fact, it gets worse, day by day, month after month. The doctor, his face dark and thoughtful, gathers the children together and, for the first time, uses the 'D' word – the one that they've all been dreading. *Dementia.* Possibly even Alzheimer's disease.

The situation slowly deteriorates; her memory loss, her confusion, her sudden bouts of agitation, her growing self-neglect, and even some occasional incontinence. The shrines of photographs lie abandoned on the shelves, dusty and disordered. Some of the porcelain statuettes have fallen off the shelves, and smashed apart. It's clear she cannot look after herself any longer. A carer is hired to live with her, and look after her throughout the day, but soon even she cannot cope. Eventually Mrs P is admitted to a specialised nursing home, many of whose residents are also elderly and demented.

Soon she can no longer recognise her own grandchildren. ('Who are they?' she mumbles, shaking her head. 'Where do they come from?') Then it's her children's turn. For a while there's still some flicker on her face whenever she hears the voice of her favourite daughter, but that too eventually fades away. When her children visit her now, she stares at them with a vague, puzzled look. She hardly speaks to anyone any more, as she shuffles silently, and a little stiffly, along the corridors of the nursing home, an aged child newly born into an unfamiliar world.

One by one her children and other relatives stop visiting her. 'What's the point?' they say to one another. 'She no longer even knows who I am.'

For the family it's a painful process, and emotionally exhausting. It seems to go on and on, without any possibility of relief. Sometimes they find themselves hoping (secretly, guiltily) that it will all end quite soon, and put an end to her suffering, and to theirs. Increasingly, they all come to regard her as already dead. 'Socially dead' as Hertz would put it, even though her body still moves and breathes, and sleeps, and regularly relieves itself. The original person no longer exists. There is no trace left behind of the woman they all once loved, the one smiling warmly back at them from all those photographs and videos – witty, intelligent, caring, always concerned for their welfare.

'I've done my mourning for her. I've grieved enough already,' says one of her daughters. 'I've already said goodbye to her,' says another. 'Actually I said it to her many months ago. I've already let go.'

And when, finally, Mrs P *does* die one day – her body this time – they are all prepared for something of an anti-climax, a mere formality. That they will have already done their mourning and crying, and said their last goodbyes, long before that final event arrives. But they are wrong. In the future there is going to be much more mourning for them to do, much more than they anticipate. They will still have to mourn for the distant past, as well as for the future that will never arrive. To grieve not only for the lost, loving mother, but also for the caring grandmother that will never again exist. Like the children of those old folks in the Home, they will discover that even a double death is not enough. There is always another stage to come.

For social death is ultimately *not* the same as a bodily death. It's only a human creation, after all. Only a pastiche of the real thing.

Each time I re-enter the Old Age Home, that building of despair, I find myself searching for some hint of life, some tiny revolt against this reversal in the natural order of deaths. That is why, on one particular visit to the Home on a summer morning, I rejoice when I'm told that one old man, 93 years old, has the habit of proposing marriage to every elderly woman who arrives in the Home. Staggering up to them with a wide, toothless smile, he sits himself down carefully beside them. A moment or so later, after some brief introductions, his old blue eyes sparkling, he takes their withered bony hand in his own and makes his romantic proposal. And each time, I'm told, his wife (also aged 90 plus) has to shuffle slowly across the room to tug him away, and to remind him, gently, that he's still a married man. And furthermore, that he's married to her. The staff tell me that each time, for a moment, he looks confused. He smiles sheepishly. Then he links his arm in hers, and they shuffle away. Forgetfulness? Confusion? An incorrigible romantic? Either way, in the warm, disinfected world of this greenhouse, filled with its doomed and muttering plants, and where every journey is racing swiftly towards death, the answer doesn't really matter.

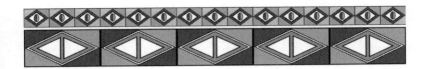

CHAPTER 10

THE APOTHEOSIS OF THE BRAIN

I t's the deepest sleep possible, one from which he will never awake. He lies quietly in the hospital room, under starched white sheets, surrounded by silent relatives and whispering nurses, and by the beep-beep-beep of the monitor machines. Gathered closely around his bed is a circle of intravenous drips, oxygen cylinders and ventilators – devices that pump air into his lungs, keep his blood flowing, and continue to infuse nutrients into his tissues. He is a youngish man, slightly unshaven, as if on the morning of the accident he was in too much of a hurry even to finish shaving. Yet he still has a good colour in his cheeks, under the heavy bandages on his head, and his body is still warm to the touch. There is even the faintest pulse, and the slow rise and fall of his chest. It is almost as if, in this depthless sleep, he was breathing all on his own. But instead of his brain directing these life-giving movements, it is machines outside his body – glistening cubes and cylinders of steel, with fluorescent dials and pulsing tubes, powered only by electricity. Machines acting as his lungs, others as his heart.

Standing at the side of the bed, the senior doctor in the long white coat slowly shakes his head, then shrugs. He says that the young man is now *brain dead*. He will never think, talk, argue, hope, imagine, dream, or remember anything ever again. The electro-encephalograph (EEG) of his brain confirms this. The senior doctor says, very emphatically, that he has a 'flat EEG', and that there is thus no electrical activity whatsoever in his brain. It is irreversibly damaged. In the words of a Dr Willard Gaylin in 1974, the young man is now a 'neomort', one of the newly dead. But thanks to the life-support machines, he is also a living cadaver, his body now ready for 'organ harvesting' – his kidneys, heart, liver, corneas and other organs all ready for removal, and then transplantation, into the grateful bodies of other people.

This unforgettable scene at a bedside – the cold finality of diagnosis. A common and tragic tableau today in many modern hospitals. But what still haunts me about it is all that focus on his *brain*, on the loss of his neurological and cognitive functions as the definitive sign of human death. Why the brain? Why the head?

It's almost as if Brain and Self were now synonymous, and that Descartes's dictum – 'I think, therefore I am' – had come true after all.

It's an old story, this focus on the head, this apotheosis of the brain. It mostly begins in the early 19th century, gathers speed in the next, and then ends up in small hospital rooms just like this one. One of its early roots was that peculiar head-based ideology, the pseudo-science called 'phrenology' – a primitive ancestor of today's neuroscience. Pioneered by two Viennese-trained physicians, Francis Gall and Johann Spurzheim, phrenology soon became widely popular throughout the USA as well as many parts of Europe.

It was based on the notion that each person's mental – as well as moral – attributes could be localised to a specific part of their brain. The actual *size* of that area was a measure of the dominance of that attribute within the individual's personality. What's more, this enlarged area was believed to correspond to an equivalent bump on the outer surface of their skull, so that by palpating the head phrenologists claimed they could identify every aspect of a personality. Long before the invention of MRI scans, they claimed that the surface of the skull – as revealed by their phrenological fingertips – was a topographical map, not only of the human mind inside it, but also of the human soul.

Gall claimed, for example, that the bump of *Poésie* was particularly prominent on the busts of famous poets, being that part of the head 'touched by the hand when composing poetry'. In the frontal eminence of the skull he could palpate the bump of Wit (*Esprit caustique*), that organ 'of the sense of the ludicrousness' so prominent, apparently, in the skulls of both Swift and Rabelais. The bump for Acquisitiveness (*Sentiment de la propriété*) was supposedly common in the pickpockets of his acquaintance.

About the same time, many early anthropologists were also focusing on the head. They were busy with callipers and measuring rules, classifying people – just like any other zoological species – into different races, based mainly on the measurements of their skulls. As the entry on 'Anthropology' in the 1875 *Encyclopaedia Britannica* puts it, 'the conformation of the skull is second only to the colour of the skin as a criterion for the distinction of races.' Having subdivided humankind in this way, they felt that they could confidently predict the moral habits, character and intelligence of any race of people. As white Europeans in an age of imperialism, they all agreed that 'the civilised white man is found to have a larger brain than the barbarian or savage.' They saw humankind as the very apex of earthly evolution, moral as well as physical. One early anthropologist, AR Wallace put it thus: 'Man is the head and culminating point of the grand design of organic nature.'

Some even claimed that the larger brain size of males meant they were superior to females; hence Charles Darwin's infamous remark about 'the less highly evolved female brain' being 'characteristic of the lower races, and therefore of a past and lower state of civilisation'.

Early natural scientists also measured animal skulls, in order to show how they differed from humans, but some of their findings made them uneasy. How to explain the uncomfortable similarity between the brain of a human and that of an ape? Their answer was that while the gorilla's brain was, admittedly, 'like a small and imperfect imitation of a man's', the crucial difference lay in the much smaller size of the primate cranium, and the less complex convolutions of the brain within it.

Almost a century later, and similar ideas formed the basis of the biological worldview and racist ideology of Nazi Germany. They too were ardent skull-measurers, and eventually the shelves of their Bureau for the Study of Ancestral Heritage were stacked with the skulls of those they regarded as members of the 'sub-human' races – many of whom, including prisoners from some concentration camps, they had murdered in the name of 'science'.

If the brain has become the site of personhood – and of all its ideas, memories, intelligence, personality and moral development – what then of the heart?

The heart was always the traditional metaphor for the Self, and for its emotions, loves, character, courage and will. Past generations regarded it as the core of a person, even as a small person in its own right. In literature, as in daily speech, hearts were said to leap, sink or jump; they broke or swelled or burst; some were large or soft, others hard or heavy or cold. For centuries people revered the sacred hearts of saints, or the romantic hearts of poets.

Perhaps the brain has replaced it because, locked in its bony box of skull, that small grey wrinkled thing has all the skills necessary for a modern industrial society: reason, calculation, logic and memory. Its apotheosis takes place in a world that now supremely values cognitive functions, rewards feats of memory, and above all emphasises the rapid storage and transmission of data – whether in a computer, or in the 'software' of the brain. A society that increasingly produces *information*, rather than goods.

Above all, the brain has come to symbolise a belief in rationality ('Use your head!'), and a passion for scientific thought. It's a potent symbol of the triumph of intellectual progress over the obscurantism of the past – of a life governed by reason and objective science, rather than by emotion or religious superstition. It can be seen as a continuation of the Enlightenment project of the late 18th century, with its view of the perfectibility of human society, and the powers of the human mind.

But there is an alternative narrative of the brain's apotheosis, especially in popular culture since the 1930s, in its magazines, books, comic strips and films. Here the brain has often been portrayed as something potentially evil and destructive. It's too much brain, and too much abstract thought, that can be so dangerous. The image of the distended, over-expanded cranium has been used to symbolise the catastrophic dangers of pure intellect, divorced from compassion and social responsibility – of a head amputated from its heart. On the lurid pages of science fiction and comic strips, there's been a whole succession of evil villains with high-domed heads – that familiar symbol of superior intelligence, and the unmistakable sign of the 'high-brow' or the 'egg-head'. Films and books portray the dangers of the 'mad scientist' or the 'evil genius' – from Dr Frankenstein up to Dr Strangelove – and his fiendish experiments, or plans for world domination. These motifs can be said to reflect a widespread fear of the consequences of science and technology run wildly out of control, with too little awareness of their impact on human life, and their effects upon the planet itself.

Recent decades have seen a phenomenal growth of interest in 'neuroscience' – the study of the structure and function of the brain, and nervous system. The US Congress declared the 1990s to be 'The Decade of the Brain', and poured many tens of millions of dollars into brain research, especially into the causes of strokes, dementias and various mental illnesses. This research has been aided by enormous advances in diagnostic technologies, such as the EEG, and CT and MRI scans.

This intense interest in brain matters has spawned a whole series of new, hyphenated sub-disciplines: *neuro*-psychiatry, *neuro*-psychology, *neuro*-pharmacology, *neuro*-ophthalmology and *neuro*-psychoanalysis (the relationship of the mind's processes to biological changes within the brain). There's even now *neuro*-theology (the study of the biological basis of religious states). Many researchers are striving to find some biological explanation, in abnormal brain structure or function, for a range of human ills, as well as social behaviour, such as criminality or drug abuse.

Scores of 'brain banks' – collections of brain and neural tissue – have been founded in different parts of the world. In 1993 the National Neurological Research Specimen Bank at the Veterans' Administration Wadsworth Hospital, University of California, Los Angeles, held more than 2000 brains, and was collecting 150 more each year. Russia, too, has been busily collecting brains. It was reported in 1991 that the Moscow Brain Institute, set up by Stalin in 1926, still had 31,000 slices of Lenin's brain, carefully preserved on microscope slides for scientific study. (One Soviet neuroscientist claimed it had an enormous number of 'giant cells' – a sign of 'superior mental function'). That same year the *New*

York Times reported that the Moscow collection of brains included those of other famous figures, such as film director Sergei Eisenstein, the writer Maxim Gorky and the poet Vladimir Mayakovsky.

The brain of Albert Einstein, removed after his death in 1955, has become one of the most famous of all human organs – revered like a potent religious relic, in a post-religious age.

Not surprisingly, in parts of the USA, there are huge fridges filled with rows of disembodied heads, shelf after shelf of them. Each one carefully labelled, they have been left in a 'cryonics' deep-freeze by their late owners in the poignant hope that one day science will somehow bring them back to life. And then perhaps allow the rest of their bodies to regenerate, from the head downwards.

Against this background is the medical concept of 'brain death', and that silent young man in the centre of a circle of life-support machines. It's only since the late 1960s that this scene has become relatively widespread. Though only a tiny percentage of deaths today, even in hospital, are actually given this diagnosis, its symbolic importance is far greater than that.

Brain death, defined as 'the permanent, irreversible ending of all electrical activity in the brain', is measured not only by an EEG but also by certain other signs, such as a deep coma, unresponsiveness to pain and lack of reflexes. Some countries have been reluctant to accept the equation of brain and person. Writing in the medical journal *The Lancet*, a Dr Nudeshima pointed out that in Japan there's been considerable cultural resistance to this Western definition of death, and to organ transplantation. This was because 'the traditional Japanese notion of person had a communal, not an individual, basis'. Death is seen there as a long process – recognised as being final only after a series of rituals conducted by the family and community – rather than as a single event. These could take weeks or even longer to complete – making it too late for any 'organ harvest'. Also, Shinto and Buddhist beliefs locate the soul everywhere in the body, not only in the brain, making it difficult to define precisely the actual moment of death. And in a society where social reciprocity is very important, some people may be resistant to receiving an organ from an anonymous donor, a person to whom they can never reciprocate; since 1999, though, this situation has been slowly changing.

The philosopher Hans Jonas has strongly criticised the Western medical definition of brain death. He sees it as a return to the old Cartesian soul-body dualism of previous centuries – only here it is replaced by the dualism of brain and body. In our more secular age, the brain becomes the new essence of the person, the new soul. This cerebral view of the self rests on the notion that 'the true human person rests in (or is represented by) the brain, of which the rest of the body is a mere subservient tool.' When the brain dies, 'it is as when the soul has departed, and all that is left are "mortal remains"' – ready to be "harvested". To Jonas, the effect of this is 'to deny the extracerebral body its essential share in the identity of the person'. 'The body is as uniquely the body of this brain and no other,' he writes, 'as the brain is uniquely the brain of this body and no other.'

But medicine has remained largely deaf to his plea. Without his, or her, brain, a person is dead – even though the rest of his body is still alive.

One day, one of my medical colleagues is called to a small, modest house in the suburbs. He's been asked to see a patient who's just been sent home from hospital. Joanna is a young woman, in her early 30s. My colleague has never met her before, but before leaving his office in the hospital, he takes a long and detailed look at the MRI scan of her head, pinning it up on a big fluorescent screen, examining it closely, inch by inch. It is a shocking picture, tragic and almost unbelievable. For most of the frontal and temporal lobes of her brain have been replaced by a ghostly, white, irregular area. He has read her medical notes carefully and knows exactly what that opaque white shape is. It is a *glioblastocytoma multiforme*, a particularly malignant form of brain tumour. He can see that it has already spread widely within her head, replacing the normal brain material until hardly any of it is left. He remembers thinking, 'How can anyone still be alive with a thing like that inside their head?' Obviously she must now be very near the end, and is probably already sunk into a deep coma, waiting for her final moment.

His visit to the house has more to do with comforting Joanna's parents, and preparing them for what is soon to come, rather than seeking to give any treatment for her condition.

He takes a deep breath, and rings the door bell. It is opened by two pale, elderly people, both of them stooped over, one holding a walking stick. They nod to him quietly, and usher him in. As he passes them in the narrow hallway, he realises that they are not elderly at all – only tired out, drained, worn away, with sunken eyes and grey, haggard, exhausted faces.

'Jo,' the old woman calls out, 'it's the doctor, Jo. He's come to see you.' The doctor cannot understand what is happening. Who is the woman talking to? Surely Joanna is deeply unconscious by now, fed only by intravenous drips, and with pale clammy skin and stertorous breathing, her face probably puckered to one side. And yet in a few moments he finds that he is completely wrong. For in the centre of the warm, stuffy bedroom, surrounded by oxygen cylinders, a commode and packets of dressings, and a small table covered with bottles of medicine, sits Joanna. She is propped up on several pillows in a wheelchair, dressed in a pink towelling dressing gown and a white nightdress decorated with tiny red flowers. She is a small shrunken woman, her face swollen and abnormally round, bloated by the steroids that she's been taking. She is quite bald, and now he notices with his sharp clinical eye the long scar on her shaven scalp, and the faint traces of blue ink criss-crossing her skull, dividing it up into different zones, and the reddened skin in each one of these from her last course of radiotherapy. And yet her blue eyes are clear, and her voice is bright, almost normal, with only a slight slurring at the edges.

'Hullo, doctor,' she says. 'I'm fine. How are you? Why are you here?'

He is amazed, quite shocked. He cannot believe it. But they talk and talk, almost as if the situation is normal. As if it were just an ordinary social encounter. The conversation is fluent, easy, without strain. And yet medically it doesn't make sense. For despite having very little brain left – at least according to the MRI scan – there is a still a person there. Someone with only a short time to live, and yet retaining a strong sense of her own self. And someone still able to smile quietly, to experience the events around her, to feel emotions, and to relate closely to other people. Even to dream a little. For when he asks her what she'd like to do in the days or weeks that remain, she replies, 'The only thing I'd like to do is see the sun setting in the countryside. To feel the warmth of it on my skin. That would make me very, very happy. That's all I want.'

Her only regret, she tells him, is that she will never have a family. And then she asks him about his own family, his only son. She asks for his name, what he looks like, his best toys and the favourite games he likes to play. She smiles a gentle, internal smile, as if his invocation of the child has given her some deep satisfaction. Almost as if that child, in some way, were her own. Gradually the doctor realises that he is beginning to relax, that she has sensed how distressed he is about her condition, and now it is *her* turn to heal him. To empathise with his pain, just as he is trying to empathise with hers.

As he leaves the house, thoughtful and subdued, but also strangely uplifted, waving goodbye to the greying couple stooped in the doorway, he is thinking about the contradiction between Joanna's disappearing brain and the survival of her strong, intact sense of herself. He knows, of course, that it will not last long, and yet already it is clear to him that a person is not merely their brain.

They are something much more than that.

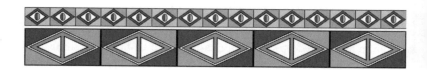

CHAPTER
11

HEARTSINK

It is just like the queue at any theatre box-office, only here it is the performers who are waiting patiently to be admitted, not the audience.

I glance around the waiting room. It's unusual for them all to come in at the same time, but today they are all here: the entire Cast. Not for the first time do I notice that they often tend to come in to the Medical Centre on the same day, even though none of them actually knows any of the others. And they also tend to come in at the busiest times, especially on a Monday morning, or else at the very last clinic late on a Friday afternoon. Afterwards they usually leave me feeling vacant, exhausted, emptied out. For each member of the Cast is one of my failures. Each one – in their own particular way – tells me a different story, and each one leaves me with feelings of defeat, frustration and often anger. Sometimes when they leave the room I feel breathless, gasping for air, as if I'd been holding my breath underwater for far too long. I'm right at the beginning of my career, and they are my 'heartsink' patients. I cannot help them no matter how hard I try. And they will not help me.

Today the Cast are mixed in with all the usual coughing, spluttering children, with their running noses or infected ears; the pregnant women gently stroking their big bellies; the old couples with hypertension or diabetes; the stroke victims with their withered limbs and irregular mouths, slumped in their chairs; the bowed-over old women with osteoporosis; and the feverish, fretful, crying babies with their tiny flushed faces.

They are all waiting to see me, some with anticipation, others with dread. The entire Cast: the Actor and the Mime, the Puppeteer, the Story-teller, the Dancer and the Opera Singer and (increasingly often these last few weeks) the Ventriloquist. All waiting to see me. Their audience of one.

Carrying my black bag I walk quickly past them, giving an occasional nod, trying not to meet anyone's eye for too long, my face frozen into a kindly, but ambiguous smile. Past the Actor, his thin lips already rehearsing his lines; past the Opera Singer, taking one sighing breath after another; past the Dancer shifting restlessly in her chair; past the Mime, his tense body gathered tightly together, as though trapped within some invisible box; past the Puppeteer, chatting quietly to several of her younger puppets; past the Story-teller frowning with concentration as she prepares her tale; and then finally past the Ventriloquist, muttering as usual to her fidgeting daughter.

I enter my consulting room. I close the door behind me and take a deep breath. The stage is ready, the props and scenery are all in place. I call for the first patient to come in. The curtain rises. My heart sinks.

The Story-teller enters the room. She is middle-aged, and faded-looking, with long straggly grey hair. She begins to speak, rapidly, breathlessly. Even before she's sat herself down across the desk from me, the words burst out of her. She says that she's feeling rather poorly, and that's why she's come in to see me today 'for a chat'. It has taken me a long time to understand how important these 'chats' are to her; how they're actually the highlight of her week, and maybe of her life. And that she's been preparing for this consultation, carefully rehearsing every detail of her story, ever since we met the week before. Today she's here, as usual, with some vague symptom or other, but really to tell me – in another short, breathless instalment – the story of her sad life. It's the one she's been narrating to me for many months now. The history of her unhappy childhood, her unhappy marriage, and her volatile relationships with each of her unhappy children. Each week some different aspect of this story emerges, always embroidered with sighs and shrugs, and long silences.

The Story-teller seems to find these sessions very satisfying.

Apparently, over many years now, she's also been seeing a series of psychotherapists, on and off. Perhaps it's because of that, but now she seems to feel that – like some sad, suburban Scheherazade – she simply *must* tell her story regularly in order to survive. Even if it takes her One Thousand and One Nights. Or even more.

Over the years, this unhappy story has been fashioned, and re-fashioned, by one doctor or therapist after another. But still her compulsion to tell it has never flagged. She *must* tell it again – to me, and to everyone else. She seems to fear the consequence of 'bottling it up', of 'not expressing' what she feels, of somehow not 'getting it off my chest'. And express it she does, again and again – sometimes only in a sequence of irregular sighs, sometimes in angry words bursting out of her like a volcanic eruption of foul pus. And yet despite all of this talking and telling and expressing, I notice how nothing really seems to change in her life. She rarely takes the advice that she is given, and rarely does she make any constructive changes. For her, it seems, the medium *is* the message. Story-telling is not a means to change, but rather a type of maintenance therapy, a life-support system in itself; like a diabetic's daily dose of insulin, or an addict's regular fix.

Mostly I feel that there's little I can do for her, except to listen. Often I resent that, especially since I have gradually begun to notice that the story she's telling me is actually taking place on two different levels. One of sighings and shrugs and muttered complaints, but the other – perhaps the more authentic one – narrated within her body, at the level of its organs, cells or chemicals. In the rising level of her blood pressure, say, the gradual clogging up of her arteries, or the increasing level of her liver enzymes – a sure sign that, despite all her denials, she's once again been drinking too much.

At the end of our talk, with me slumped exhausted in my chair, she leaves the room. Nothing has changed, of course, except that now she looks relieved, relaxed.

At least, until her next appointment.

Marcel the Mime, by contrast, is a man of very few words. He is pale, withdrawn, taciturn, and sometimes seems almost to be mute. He hardly ever complains, hardly ever admits that he is ill or suffering or unhappy. He downplays every illness, minimises every bodily malfunction. Mostly silent and hunched over, with a pale morose face, he shuffles slowly from the doorway to the chair placed near to my desk. Today, as usual, he has come in to see me with some minor complaint. I know that nothing serious will be found, and yet once more I feel that he is actually 'talking' to me in a very different, but silent language. It is a complex sign language that I've never been able to decode. A language of grimaces and postures, of frowns or sighs, a deep shrug or two, a slumped shoulder, a nervous tic, a tremor, even an occasional smile, sometimes subtle changes of behaviour or clothing. Each time Marcel says very little, and yet his body speaks loudly instead.

Sometimes, and for no apparent reason, he begins to attend the Medical Centre much too often, but sometimes not often enough. On many occasions he misses his appointments, and I see the letters 'DNA' ('Did Not Arrive') scrawled irritably in his medical file by one of the receptionists. At other times, he comes in too often, becoming, at least for a while, what doctors disparagingly call a 'frequent attender'. But all this time he says virtually nothing. He is monosyllabic, withdrawn, evasive. He never reveals what is truly bothering him. I guess he is lonely and sad, with many personal problems, and probably feels undervalued and underpaid, but those are merely my hunches. Marcel never admits to anything.

But there are times, very occasionally, when I think I'm beginning to understand what he is silently trying to 'say'. To decode the Rosetta Stone of his suffering, and the message he so subtly encodes within his symptoms: a chest pain standing in, perhaps, for a broken heart; a headache for some unpleasant thought; an abdominal pain for bad news that he simply cannot digest. But my relief at this new clarity soon vanishes. For when I suggest this to him, he still says nothing, admits to nothing. His presence becomes even more of an absence than it was before. No matter what I do or say, when he leaves the room I am always left wondering: What is Marcel *really* trying to say?

With Harvey, the Actor, it's just as difficult to make a diagnosis. But the reasons for this are very different. His story is always confusing. Is he really in *so* much pain, or is he not? Is that man sitting opposite me, moaning and sobbing and gripping his stomach so tightly (last week it was his chest, the week before his back), really as ill as he appears to be? And now he is pointing, with a shaking finger, at a tiny blemish, a mere bump on his arm, convinced that he has cancer, and is about to die. Again, I can find nothing wrong. 'Oh!-Oh!-Oh!' he moans, as I try to examine him, 'Oh!-Oh!-Oh!'

Maybe after all, Harvey is merely a hypochondriac, but if so he has learned his lines very well from doctors, as well as from television. He has learnt how to confuse me, and every other doctor that he meets. For his story is always plausible and convincing. And it always leaves me worried that I am missing something – the *real* diagnosis. I've learned that he's addicted to television soap operas set in medical practices or in hospitals, especially American hospitals. I know he loves the drama of those films, the green-clad doctors rushing along the corridors, pushing along those gurneys of broken, bleeding people, bursting through the swing doors into the Emergency Room. He loves the beautiful nurses, the soulful, handsome doctors, the weeping, terrified, tragic patients. He seems to have decided that if he cannot become one of those doctors, then at least he can be one of their patients. But he still leaves me feeling anxious.

Each time I see him, his voice is loud and booming. It projects right across my desk; it seems to fill the room. Last week he was Hamlet – melancholy, indecisive, uncertain about his fate. The week before he was Macbeth – bold, assertive, demanding, focused on his future, and on the medical treatment that he required. Today he is portraying someone else. But whom? He sobs, sighs, rolls his eyes, grips his head or his tummy or chest, grimaces, moans, shifts uneasily around in his chair. His descriptions of his symptoms are always florid. He uses vivid words to describe them: 'I felt so bad when I had the 'flu,' he says, 'that I almost *died*!' 'That migraine attack last week *almost killed* me!' The pains that he suffers from are always *excruciating*; he always feels *utterly exhausted*; his feelings of anxiety are always *intolerable*; a minor cold makes him feel *totally debilitated*; with backache he can *hardly move*. I think of him as some out-of-work thespian, desperately over-acting at an audition, but he still leaves behind the question: what is he really trying to *say*? Is he really in *so* much discomfort? And, in that case, have I somehow missed some vital diagnostic clue – even though his medical tests are all negative? These questions remain hovering in the air, like the faint echo of applause, long after he has left my room, bowing slightly, always smiling, my prescription gripped tightly in his hand.

And they are questions I ask myself, again and again. Even in the early hours of the morning, as I toss and turn, I am still asking them.

Madeleine, the Opera Singer, is plump and Rubensesque, with a large expansive bosom. Like some sad suburban diva, whenever I see her she is singing some lonely and irritating song. Her voice is loud and expansive, but also tremulous at the edges. Each time she enters my room, she seems to expand to fill it, every crevice of it, with her ample bosom and her high soprano voice, her emphatic gestures and poses, her big rings and earrings, her bright flamboyant clothes. She is much like the Actor, only louder, and much more passionate. But unlike him, Madeleine never performs alone. She always needs some chorus in the background, a supporting cast, or the sounds of an orchestra swelling in counterpoint to her shrill, complaining voice. I guess she would prefer something that grandiose, of course, but in the meantime she has to make do with the background murmur from the crowded waiting room, the clink of medical instruments, the compassionate tut-tut of her young doctor, the sympathetic clucking of one of her children, or the murmured solicitations of her tiny husband – a miniature man, dapper in blue blazer and bow-tie, with a soft beard and a worried face.

Whenever she leaves my room, the sounds of her last aria still ringing in my ears, it feels all silent and empty. It is like the atmosphere in a theatre after the applause have died away, the emptying seats strewn with discarded programmes, the curtains tightly drawn, the stage deserted. And always I am left wondering at my own dry mouth and exhausted voice, and the ache in my shoulders and arms. As if I too have been applauding too vigorously, and for far too long.

Now the Dancer enters the room, sweeping towards me in her red scarf and woollen leg-warmers, her pashmina thrown hurriedly over her shoulders. She seldom seems to walk, only to fly, to leap through the air from one place to another. She is always on the move, always in a hurry, never at rest. In her personal life, too, the Dancer always moves quickly, whirling, swirling, pirouetting from one marriage to another. Each of these marriages seems like a different type of dance: a samba or salsa with one young man, then a slow and decorous waltz with an older one, then a lambada with that wild waiter she met on holiday, and finally a volatile tango with her present spouse. And now she sits impatiently across the desk from me, glancing repeatedly at her watch, shifting restlessly in her chair. As always she appears to be anxious to move away, to fly, to leave this consultation quickly behind her. She is always in motion, travelling here, rushing to an appointment there. She makes me nervous, for sometimes all I can see of her is a multi-coloured blur seated before me, or a type of kinetic flash at the very periphery of my vision.

Gradually I've come to realise that she is not dancing towards any destination. Rather, she is dancing *away* from something. It is something quite terrible, I gather, though I have never learnt exactly what. Probably some depthless depression, a terror of some sort, that waits in ambush for her, and always has done so, ever since she was a child – but I am never sure. Sitting in that chair, I see a moving, restless, impatient body, a body that seems always to be in motion, always balancing on its toes, always half-here and yet not-here. Always fleeing from itself. Yet there's just no way to stop her dance, or to somehow slow her down, although I've tried again and again. Despite my efforts, it seems important for her that the show must go on. And on. And so it will do, I suppose. Until at last her final and inevitable solo performance takes place in an Intensive Care Unit somewhere, or in one of the wards of the local psychiatric hospital.

It's the turn of the Puppeteer. Maria always comes into the consulting room with one or more of her daughters, or sometimes a granddaughter or two. As always, I notice how she sits silently at the centre of a circle of sad, silent young women, some resting their hands on her shoulders, others gently stroking her hair. Very occasionally they seem bored or resentful, but mostly they just look anxious and pale. Maria is a living example of the Spanish saying, *mujer infirma, mujer eternal* – a sick mother lives forever. For decades now, I gather, her suffering and symptoms, her unhappiness and many disappointments, have been the central drama of her family's life. 'What can we do about mother?' has been the recurrent question for most of their lives. It has caused quarrels among the sisters, or between them and their husbands. *'What can we do about mother?'* And everything has got much worse since her husband died; even deeper sighs, and an even wider circle of different daughters, or restless grandchildren, who orbit around her like worried planets. Gathered in an anxious clump in my room, they usually do all the talking. 'My mother isn't feeling well today,' they say, or 'My mother is feeling rather faint,' or 'The tablets you gave my mother aren't helping her very much.'

Maria herself says hardly anything, only sits quietly at the hub of all this attention, sighing and shaking her head, and sometimes wiping away an invisible tear. But for all her apparent detachment, I've noticed how fully alert she is. How subtly and with only the tiniest gesture or sigh, she tugs occasionally on an invisible string, manipulating her puppets carefully, and skilfully, one by one. Soon I, too, find myself ensnared in her strings, until I can hardly move or breathe. There is no point in struggling. I find myself agreeing with almost everything she says. I write out all the prescriptions that she wants, give her the referral letters that she asks for. There is nothing I can say to interrupt the show. Nothing, it seems, can ever cut those powerful strings, or halt the performance halfway through.

Finally, it's time for the Ventriloquist. She is the one who affects me most of all, who leaves me feeling most defeated. She is in her late 40s, or early 50s, with an upper-class accent and manner, always smartly dressed, with silver bracelets and expensive pearls, her hair carefully coiffured. And yet, if only I was more observant, or more experienced, I would spot the cracks in that mask. The ones I somehow choose to ignore, until it is much too late. The fissures in her face powder; the smeared mascara; the dark glasses she always wears, even indoors; the agitated tremor lurking in her voice; the nicotine stains on each of her perfumed fingertips.

She comes in as usual with one of her children. This one, Fiona, is about 13 – a pale, delicate child with a sensitive face and curly blond hair. She sits staring at the floor, silent and passive, sometimes fidgeting a little. The Ventriloquist launches into her usual speech. She says that she is worried about her daughter. She says that Fiona is 'uncooperative' and 'naughty' and 'disobedient'. Her behaviour is mischievous and difficult. She is often moody, doesn't sleep well at night, and often has headaches or tummy pains. She has even, on one occasion, wet her bed (here the child becomes more restless, chewing at her lower lip). Her mother says that because all her medical tests were negative, Fiona is clearly unwell in another way. An emotional way. And she cannot cope with her behaviour any longer. She simply *cannot* cope. She demands of me, her voice hard and rising fast, that I send her daughter to a psychiatrist, or even a psychologist, 'for treatment'. And *soon*. She says that Fiona needs 'proper professional help' – but certainly not from me; too young, too inexperienced, and with that broad colonial accent. She needs someone who can treat her daughter 'professionally', and make her behaviour more 'normal'.

Each time I ask Fiona what she thinks about it all, she answers quietly, her voice faint and whispering. She says that she agrees with everything her mother has said. It seems that I have no choice. I write the letter.

Only much later (but unfortunately too late for Fiona) do I learn, with growing unease, that in family therapy Fiona would be termed the 'Identified Patient', or else the 'Symptom Carrier'. She would be seen as perhaps the healthiest person in a very sick family. The lightning conductor, the scapegoat, the one onto whom all the family pathology is projected. For it is the Ventriloquist who is emotionally unwell, and very deeply so, not her children. She is the one who needs professional help, though of course she will never accept it. In the meantime, week after week, it is her own anguish that 'speaks' to the doctor – indirectly, and through the suffering bodies and psyches of her children. They are carrying her symptoms, mouthing her words.

And in my youthful inexperience, I am her accomplice. Whenever she leaves the room it is not only the usual exasperation that I feel. It is also guilt.

In the secret bestiary of any group of doctors, people like the Cast are known as 'heartsink' patients. And for good reason. For even when there are only a few of them around, they cause their doctors both an enormous amount of stress, and a high proportion of their workload. One textbook defines them, in a careful understatement, by their 'highly complex and often multiple problems (some real, others not): and [by the] exasperation generated between patient and doctor'. It also lists some of the 'risk factors' of the doctors that deal with them: their lack of training in counselling skills, and the burden of an unreasonably high workload. In my early years in clinical practice, both apply to me.

The psychiatrist Michael Balint, in his book *The Doctor, The Patient and the Illness*, has described many of these people, and the effects that they can have on their doctors. He writes about the types of families that they come from, and the intricate patterns of relationships that may produce or sustain their behaviour. Many not only present with puzzling, inexplicable symptoms – they are also 'nomads', constantly shifting their allegiance from one doctor to another, or wandering endlessly among different hospitals. They are the ones who always seem to be angry and dissatisfied with their doctor's treatment and yet, oddly, many of them return to consult that same doctor, with the same symptoms, time after time. Despite the fact that no treatment seems to work for them. No medicine ever relieves their symptoms. No advice given is ever taken. 'Why don't you...' suggests the doctor each time; 'Yes, *but...*' they always reply.

Balint suggests that people like this often choose their doctors (or remain with them) to satisfy some special psychological need. On a deep level these needs may actually match those of their doctor's, in an unconscious collusion of unhealthy traits. On one side of the desk, a need to suffer and never to be helped – and on the other side, a need to feel helpless and inadequate.

The wounding power of heartsinks is a by-product also of the doctor's own *déformation professionelle*: their need to be needed, to cure, to have power over disease, and some control over human suffering. But also of their delusion that there is always some medical 'quick fix' for human misfortune, a pill for every personal problem. Perhaps it's because of this that you won't find the members of the Cast described in detail in any medical textbook, and only occasionally hinted at in an indirect way. They're always the unwelcome ghosts at the celebratory feasts of medical science. The failures of treatment, the one's who got away.

No-one at medical school ever told me about them. No-one ever advised me how to deal with them, or with my own reactions to them. They were regarded merely as an irritant, an embarrassment – as pieces of grit in the otherwise smoothly working machine of medical diagnosis and treatment.

But I've come to see them rather differently. And to regard them not just as a problem, but also as the occasional bearers of a rare gift. For they can sometimes bring with them both insights and self-awareness for their doctor. They can tell him (or her) a lot about himself, his deepest anxieties, the chinks in his psychological armour. Occasionally, and for just one awful moment, they can even remind him of himself, offer him a glimpse of his own fractured reflection in the pieces of a broken mirror – evoking old memories, perhaps, like the echo of a depressed mother's voice, or the judgemental tone of an angry father. And a tiny minority of these heartsink patients (but always the most virulent of all) seem to sense this. Their antennae are sensitive and ever keen. They sense their doctor's vulnerabilities. They become experts, probably unconsciously, in scraping the scabs off those ancient wounds. Like sharks or piranha fish, the worst of them are fatally attracted to the presence of blood.

Like every other form of healing, medicine is a form of theatre, a very special type of performance. To be successful it needs a precise choreography. It needs its props and scenery and costumes, its particular smells, and special words said by the healer in a very special way. All of this helps to create a particular atmosphere, to enhance the authority of the healer, and the trust of those who consult them. Both parties play the roles, often unconsciously, according to society's expectations. The script tells patients how to display their suffering, and doctors how to react. It provides tacit rules on how to behave, speak and act during the encounter. What should be said, and what should be left out.

On the tiny stage of the clinic or the ward, both patient and practitioner give their special performances. It is not only the intersection of two formalised roles, scripted long in advance. It is also a duet, a *pas de deux*.

As the solitary spectator huddled helplessly in my chair, watching all of this – one performance after another, every day of the week – I often reflect on how we over-value words. How 'talk therapy' has become such a common way for people to express their unhappiness, resolve their conflicts, or even gain absolution. And yet words are only one form of expression, for the members of the Cast express their suffering in different forms, act out their scripts in very different ways. Each has their own dialect of distress. Dealing with them involves recognising early on what dialect they are using at that particular moment, out of the vast Babel of possibilities – even if, apparently, they are saying nothing at all.

Sometimes, in my little theatre, lined with textbooks and medical instruments, I find myself wishing for a very different type of performance. Desperately hoping that the Opera Singers would turn silently into Mimes; or the Mimes would begin to articulate their problems a little more clearly; or that the Actors would sometimes mime a little more, and speak a little less; or that the Dancers would stop their frenzied flight from here to there, and rest for a while; or that the Puppeteers would cut the strings of their poor marionettes, and let them go free; or that the Ventriloquists would stop their ... But then I remind myself that it's often all about the performance itself. For some, apparently, that's what gives them most satisfaction, and that's where any healing really takes place – even if the effect is only temporary. It's their chance to perform from their very own script – a role that they've mastered over many years, and are reluctant to abandon. It's their ritual of healing, their own way of making themselves feel better. And here the doctor's role is mainly to provide a safe space in which all those different styles of performance can take place. And then to watch and to listen and nod occasionally, and accept (often very reluctantly) the passive role of audience. But at the same time always acknowledging, whether openly or not, the pain and the anxiety that usually lie hidden behind the costumes, the masks, and the thick layers of make-up.

In any case, after the show is over, the performers rarely leave the room empty-handed. Instead of a round of applause, a bouquet of roses, an Oscar or a fat cheque, they usually leave with some reassurance, and the satisfying sense of actually having been seen or heard. Even sometimes with a prescription clutched tightly in a sweating hand, or – most prized of all – a referral letter to the top medical specialist in town.

It seems that there are times in medical practice (fortunately only a few) when you simply cannot cure, and you cannot heal. When there is absolutely nothing that you can do to change a person's situation, or to alter their behaviour. It's the wisdom of knowing when to do *less*, as well as when to do more. Despite what the textbooks say, with people like those in the Cast (with the possible exception of the Ventriloquist and the Puppeteer), it means seeing one's medical role in a different way. It means accepting the limitations of medicine, and the fact that there are times when all one can do is sit back and watch, and listen closely, and bear compassionate witness as the long cavalcade of human suffering passes slowly before you.

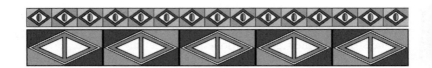

CHAPTER 12

WOUNDED HEALERS

The room is icy and tense, with tiled walls and long opaque windows. Today as usual it is crowded with white-coated medical students sitting in a semi-circle around a silent, naked figure lying on a long metal table. Standing besides it is our lecturer in a white rubber apron and boots, and wearing white rubber gloves. There's no need for him to wear a mask at this operation, for this particular patient is not in any danger of infection. Suddenly the lecturer lifts up his scalpel. The buzz of conversation in the room dies quickly away. The autopsy is about to begin.

We are in our third year of studies at the University of Cape Town Medical School. The bodies that our lecturer examines are brought down every day from Groote Schuur Hospital, up on the hill. Usually they are the wrecked, archaeological remains of elderly patients who have died on the wards. Every week we find them lying on the metal table before us; thin, silent, alabaster figures with collapsed mouths and empty, staring eyes, like statues discarded by their sculptor. Sometimes on a body's surface, there's a reminder of the medical treatment they had undergone right at the very end – a fresh unhealed surgical scar; a needle from an intravenous drip still left in a vein; a bandage; a dressing. But inside those pale bodies, the pathologist's scalpel reveals a very different world – a complex and multi-coloured one, with knots of shiny organs and blood vessels, nerves, ligaments, and bones, all emerging from their hiding places beneath the skin. They are soft and friable and strangely coloured, and as they spill out of the body onto the metal tray they don't resemble at all the bright illustrations in my anatomy textbook. The liver is black and jelly-like, soft and slippery, like the ones glimpsed in a butcher's shop, rather than in the pages of any book. The brain, which he removes after cutting noisily through the skull with an electric saw, before placing it in an enamel basin before us, is all grey and wrinkled, and resembles nothing more than an aging scrotum.

The pathologist examines each organ carefully, weighs it, and then makes detailed notes of what he finds. Sometimes he removes slices for microscopic examination, or else fills test tubes with samples of various body fluids. All of these will be tested in the laboratory, in order to identify the exact cause of the person's death. And then there is that smell – the one I can never quite remember, but somehow can never quite forget. A sour, sharp smell that rises out of those ruined abdomens, vacant chests and empty heads, and drifts uneasily around the crowded room.

One day when we take our seats, we find a 'fresh cadaver' lying on the long metal table. But this one is different from all the others we have seen so far. It is the one that I can never forget. He is a young man with sunken cheeks and dark hair, and seems to be only a few years older than we are. He is tanned and slightly unshaven, his eyes closed, as though he were just taking a nap after a long day spent on Muizenberg beach, swimming or surfing, and the faint flush of life seems still to linger on his cheeks. He must have died that morning, or yesterday at the very latest. The pathologist is in good form today, amiable and informative, and full of anecdotes about difficult autopsies he's done in the past. As usual, he hardly glances towards us, as he busies himself in preparation. Then, without delay or warning, he leans forward and hollows the young man out, dismantles him, takes him apart only a few feet away from us, all the while chatting away, even telling the occasional wry joke, as he pulls from the man's abdominal cavity the pale, odiferous coils of his small intestine (their surfaces speckled, I notice, with multiple tiny haemorrhages). Then, in the shocked silence, saws open the thorax, removes the heart and lungs from their attachments – the bronchi, the thoracic aorta, the superior vena cava, and all the rest – pulls them out of the body, and throws them heavily into the enamel basin nearby. They fall into it with a moist, slapping, squishing sound. Then, still talking mainly to himself, he noisily saws open the skull, pulls out the brain, and tosses it into the basin with the rest. There is a shocked silence in the room. Many have stopped writing. There is only the dripping of taps, the clank of instruments, the drone of the pathologist's voice.

A quarter of an hour or so later (though it seems much longer) he has finished his dissection. Emptied of organs, the vacant space within the young man's body is replaced by sawdust, before it is sewn up again. The students get up silently, and begin to file out of the room. For an awful moment those words of TS Eliot in *The Waste Land* come back to me, with a terrible resonance: 'We are the hollow men, we are the stuffed men.' In this icy little room, those words seem to have a special relevance.

Not for the first time do I wonder whether, after all these shocking experiences at medical school, we too have been emptied out, and then our insides filled up again with a very different stuff.

That night I can hardly sleep, again. I have those nightmares, the ones about disintegration, like those I used to have the previous year after dissecting cadavers in the Anatomy Department. All that slow dismantling of pale wasted figures lying on their stone slabs, each one swaddled in damp cloth like an ancient mummy. The sharp, sour smell of formaldehyde, the low murmur of voices, the chilly air. Once more now the world seems to me to have been turned upside-down, inside-out. And then taken apart. Everything is reversed, for what should have been together, is now apart. What is usually inside, is now outside. In the name of medical science, a human body much like ours has been violated, and there was nothing we could do to stop it.

Two years later and we are at the police mortuary in Salt River, a smaller, much tenser crowd of students this time. The policemen at the reception desk stare at us suspiciously, and then enter our names carefully, one by one, into a big ledger. In this mortuary, unlike at the hospital, the bodies are all casualties – people who have died violently, unnaturally and well before their time. Today there's to be an autopsy on what little remains of an African man, incinerated in a shack fire on the windy Cape Flats. And another one on an African woman, stabbed to death, maybe in the same shantytown. And then there's a newly born baby, found abandoned on a rubbish dump. And finally, at the end of the morning, an autopsy on the body of a coloured prisoner, punctured by a bullet wound, and apparently shot while trying to escape. Throughout the procedure, a uniformed prison officer with a big red face, shaven head and khaki uniform stands silently besides the autopsy tray, as though the prisoner might try to escape yet again. Occasionally glaring at us or at the pathologist, he is making copious notes in a large black book. He makes us nervous. He makes us want to escape, but also frightened to do so.

I'm not the only one who finds it increasingly difficult to attend these autopsies, whether at Salt River or at the medical school. Many of my fellow students make excuses not to attend, developing sudden coughs or inexplicable fevers. Others get their friends to forge their signatures on the attendance register. Some, like me, retreat into dreams – or into nightmares.

Years later and the smell of those autopsies still mingles in my mind with the smoke from the tall crematorium chimney beside it. It is a sweet, uneasy smell, carried by the wild Cape winds through the windows of the student residence, drifting along the corridors and then into my room, infiltrating my mind with its dark message. It mingles with the incense that I burn to dispel it, and with the faint tang of formaldehyde that clings to my dissecting kit. And sometimes with that confident, plastic smell that rises from the glossy pages of my big American textbooks.

Every day, death and dying in the wards, death described in detail in our lectures, and then death minutely dissected in the autopsy room. Death is so omnipresent that sometimes I feel a dark tide of despair rising within me. To keep it at bay I find myself searching vainly for some sense of beauty, for a small elusive zone of peace and solace among all this destruction. Some space that is still pure and uncontaminated by human suffering. Most Sunday nights I go to concerts at the Cape Town City Hall. On weekends I attend art exhibitions in town, visit friends, climb Lion's Head, or sunbathe on Clifton Beach, but all this doesn't really clear my mind. For back at the medical school on Monday mornings those same cells still stare up at me from the microscope slide, with their pinkish cytoplasm, and their large dark irregular nuclei, like the pupils of extra-terrestrial eyes. In a perverse, terrible way those cancer cells on the slide have a certain cruel beauty about them in all their chaotic profusion, as if they were bouquets of brightly petalled flowers, piled high at a funeral.

'So you've also noticed that?' a friend says to me guiltily one day, avoiding my eye, and then we quickly change the subject and never mention it again.

Then after graduation there are the intense years of internship, and beyond, working in different hospitals in various departments: medicine, paediatrics, surgery, orthopaedics. Long nights without sleep, roaming the darkened wards filled with coughs and troubled breathing, of whimpers and low moans from the restless lines of shadowy shapes on either side of the ward, among the low beep-beep of the monitor machines. Sometimes small intense clumps of doctors and nurses are gathered around a particular half-lit bed, trying desperately to resuscitate a dying person. At other beds, they are slowly drawing the sheets over someone's pale, silent face. There is a constant sense of exhaustion, running between wards and clinics from one sudden emergency to another. And there's that pervasive anxiety about making a mistake: the wrong diagnosis, the wrong dose of medication.

One night in a paediatric ward a baby dies gasping in my arms as we desperately try to revive it, while the nurses scream for the paediatrician, busy in another part of the building. In internal medicine, an old man dies sighing in the ward, and the nurse standing beside me suddenly becomes hysterical, sobbing into her hands, then biting at her clenched fists. The old man, it turns out, was her father, but until that moment she had kept that secret from everyone. No-one knew, until it was much too late, and I never knew why. Then, in another ward a young girl, about our own age, bald, pale from chemotherapy, is slowly consumed by leukaemia. We watch her fading away, day by day. Each day a little thinner, her voice a little fainter. We can do nothing to help her.

Memory after memory, a whole multi-coloured library of them. Nightmares and daydreams and flashbacks, crowding into my head, taking up residence forever just inside my eyelids.

Some of us are storing up these traumas – a reservoir of dangerous memories that will one day re-emerge like a time-bomb, at quite unexpected times. In the meantime some of my colleagues flee into alcohol, others into sex, drugs, or even sport. Some never make it through the year. We are like those other young doctors so vividly described in Samuel Shem's novel *The House of God*, with their breakdowns, alcoholism, marital problems and drug abuse. Many of us – though not all – will emerge from all these many experiences as wounded healers. Elated about having become *real* doctors at last but also, on some level, deeply scarred.

Medical training can be a traumatic time, but it's usually more so than it need be. I've often puzzled about why this should be so. But it's only when studying anthropology, shortly after medical school, that the connection becomes clear. Was there a link between this type of training and the training of other forms of healer found elsewhere, in more traditional societies? At first the idea seems fanciful, but then I begin to wonder whether all that suffering inflicted on medical students and young doctors may *not* be entirely accidental. Not just a matter of a massive workload, lack of sleep, poor staffing and inadequate resources, but on some level quite deliberate. A type of initiation process, a primitive rite of passage into an esoteric and guarded profession – what anthropologists sometimes call a 'curative cult'. In order to become a healer, it may well be essential to become wounded in some way. And if that's the case, then maybe it's not always such a bad thing.

In many of the groups of healers found worldwide, each member has been wounded in some way – either before their training, or during their initiation. Becoming a member is a harsh endurance test, a means of strengthening them for the challenges to come. In a medical education, exposing you early on to traumatic experiences means preparing you for the endless procession of disease and death that you will inevitably encounter, and thus making it easier for you to cope. But for some people, those same wounds designed to protect them, may have exactly the opposite effect. They may even destroy them

I think of my father, a consultant psychiatrist in South African state hospitals, and more especially of some of his colleagues. Many of them are strained, exhausted men and women, with grey frowning faces and tobacco-stained fingertips. Some of them drink too much, or drive too fast. Others get divorced much too often. Depression and even suicide stalk some of them like predators. They are over-stressed, damaged people working at the very frontline of health care, paying a heavy price – as many doctors always do – for acting as the delicate membrane between hope and despair, life and death. For feeling the pain of others, while ignoring their own. For their specific job is not only to treat patients, but also to act as a human barrier between 'normal' society and all those chaotic people that society can never accept. Whatever the risk to themselves, they must stand, firmly between the two Janus faces of all human life: Order and Chaos.

There seems to be one particular type of traditional healer that's most relevant for this comparison. It is the *shaman*, a figure who appears in different forms in most traditional cultures. These are people who, under certain circumstances, are believed to 'incarnate' certain malevolent spirits within themselves, in order to control them. For that reason the shaman is sometimes known as a 'master of spirits', because in this state of possession (a trance, or some other altered state of consciousness) he (or she) can then use these spirits to diagnose and treat other people – especially those afflicted by those same malevolent spirits. Like the recovering alcoholics in an Alcoholics Anonymous group, their past problems help to sensitise them to these same problems in others, and so make it easier to help them. Some form a group of healers that anthropologists would call a 'community of suffering'.

Becoming a shaman is a long and arduous process. Often it is dangerous to both body and mind. It frequently begins with a major crisis: a severe illness, a major injury, a 'nervous breakdown', even a psychotic episode. To the neophyte shaman, newly possessed by spirits, and facing the struggle to master these powerful and destructive forces, it can feel as though he is near to death. The anthropologist Piers Vitebsky describes how, in Mongolia and Siberia, for example, the first approach by the spirits is in the form of a violent onslaught – an intense form of emotional and physical suffering, that seems to shatter the shaman's personality, or even his body. Young shamans often have dreams or visions of their body being dismantled, dismembered, taken apart by the spirits. In parts of Asia and the Americas, they may even feel themselves being stripped down to a skeleton. For the trainee shaman it is a time of chaos and confusion. In terrifying dreams of dismemberment, the spirits cut up their bodies, dissect them, remove the limbs, rip out the organs, break open the skull. Later on in the trance, or in their training, they will be re-assembled and re-born, put together again: bones will be joined to bones, joints reconstituted, organs replaced, flesh and muscles added, and all of this enclosed once more in its envelope of skin.

Eventually the crisis will be over. The shaman will emerge from it deeply changed, and with a very different view of the world. He (or she) returns to everyday life ready now to heal those still afflicted by those same spirits. His painful experience of death and re-birth has healed him. He is wounded, but those wounds have brought him greater wisdom, a deeper understanding of human suffering.

Doctors, of course, are not shamans. They are scientists, and as such are coming from a very different place. But they are also healers of a sort, or at least should be, and not just technicians of the body. And like this other form of healer they, too, are dismantled during their training, but it's done indirectly. One stage at a time, and in slow motion over several years. I think of that year in the dissecting room, taking apart a human form, dismembering it, pulling out its faded organs, cutting off its limbs, sawing open its skull. During that year, and later in the autopsy room, it felt as if we were somehow breaking some ancient taboo, dismantling with our scalpels and saws some ancient sense of what it means to be human. And perhaps deep down, by dismantling the human forms before us, we are also, in some sense, dismantling ourselves.

Later on in busy clinical practice, our struggle will not only be to reassemble ourselves, and our patients, from all of these scattered fragments. It will also be to control our own feelings and fears, and all those painful memories – much as a shaman might struggle to control the malevolent spirits that possess him – in order to use those experiences to heal others. It seems to be a necessary stage in becoming a doctor. Another type of wounded healer.

I am very new to clinical practice, as well as to England, when I am suddenly called to a large suburban house to see a middle-aged man. 'My husband's got a pain in his leg,' says his wife's breathless voice on the telephone. 'Actually, it's in both his legs.' I read through his medical notes before I leave the Medical Centre. There is almost nothing significant in them. The man is affluent and well educated. He appears to be quite healthy for his age, except for his diabetes, and that has seemingly been well controlled – or at least it was so, several years ago, when he last consulted a doctor. For some odd reason, he's not attended the Medical Centre since then. So presumably he's still OK.

It is one of the neatest gardens I have ever seen, in one of the neatest suburbs around. The hedge in front of the house is tightly coiffured, every bush and shrub has been neatly trimmed, every flower carefully pruned, every fallen leaf carefully removed. The small patch of grass in front has been mown so closely that it now resembles a green carpet more than a lawn. Besides it are neat rectangular beds of geraniums, with a carefully shaped buddleia in the background, while on either side of the central pathway, with its symmetrical paving stones arranged in a perfect geometric design, stand rigid rows of potted ferns, like soldiers on parade. Just in front of the varnished front door, with its shiny brass door knocker, is a tiny bower of clematis and climbing roses, also carefully trimmed. The house seems brand new, almost as if it's just been delivered straight from a glossy catalogue. The paintwork is perfect, the windows seem newly polished, the window sills carefully scrubbed.

When she opens the door, I see that Mrs R is exactly like her garden. Her hair, like her hedges, has been carefully groomed, her eyebrows neatly plucked above an immaculate mask of face powder. And yet there is something about her face – maybe the slightly reddened eyes, the sag of those carefully made-up cheeks, the faintest twitch of a lipsticked mouth – that doesn't quite fit. Something is out of place. It's as if a painting had been placed, quite inadvertently, within entirely the wrong sort of frame.

She nods and stands aside to let me in. 'Sorry to call you out, doctor,' she says. 'I know you're very busy. My husband's upstairs. His legs are hurting him, but I'm sure it's nothing serious. Just a little infection or something. He always makes such a fuss about everything. You know what men are like.'

The entrance hall and the sitting room are just as immaculate – white walls, a spotless dining suite, a suite of comfortable chairs in cream-coloured leather. But that *smell!* For woven into the usual bouquet of suburbia – floor polish, air fresheners, detergents, and Mrs R's own perfume – is something else which at first I cannot identify, but which gets stronger as I climb the stairs. I struggle to remember. Surely it cannot be... I have not experienced anything like that ever since I was a medical student in Cape Town, years before. Surely not *here*, in London. In an affluent suburb? It just cannot be. The smell is intimate and horrifying and, as I climb the stairs, increasingly familiar.

I had completely forgotten it, and even forgotten that I'd once experienced it. The memory of that incident had been buried I had hoped – with so many others – somewhere deep underground. But sour and sickly, that smell now takes me back and back to another time. It is Cape Town in the 1960s, and a poor coloured man is lying in a hospital bed. He has just been admitted to the ward. He has ragged clothes, a pale unshaven face and missing front teeth, some faded tattoos and a long scar across his scalp. He has heart trouble and advanced diabetes, and has been an alcoholic for very many years. And a heavy smoker, too, whenever he can afford it. Now after an injury to his leg, which he never brought for treatment before, he is lying there, smiling up at us in a confused and irregular way. He is feverish, almost delirious. He is very close to death. And that powerful, troubling smell is rising around him from his lower body. Someone lifts up the hospital blanket, and removes the temporary dressing. I have to stop myself gagging. It is horrific, this wreck that was once a man, destroyed so totally by poverty and disease and neglect. Others quickly cover their noses and mouths with sleeves or handkerchiefs. There it is – gangrene. That rotting, oozing, fungating leg, dark greenish and mottled almost up to his knee, bordered by inflamed skin, the blackened toes, the foot and lower leg half dropping off. It's a death sentence, one that will be carried out, only an hour or so later.

Back in the suburban house, I look at the man in the bed again. But unlike that man back in Cape Town he is well off and well educated, and it's clear that he's been like this for days, or more likely for weeks. And yet all that time they have done nothing. Never lifted up the telephone, never dialled the doctor. Now his condition is too far gone. Most of the toes are involved on both feet, and part of the foot on one side. The smell is overpowering. I resist the instinct to cover my face, hide my nose in my sleeve. Despite the drizzle and the unfamiliar streets outside, all those African memories are flooding back again. The ones I had long forgotten. Now raw chaos is bursting out here, in suburban London, in the middle of all this bourgeois calm. Chaos inside myself, as well as in the bed before me. The woman's shoulders are shaking now, her mask of face powder beginning to dissolve like a dry riverbed caught in a heavy rainstorm. She is sobbing and sobbing, but the man says nothing.

There's no need to scold them for the delay. There's no point. For I know that soon much more will be amputated from their lives than just a blackened foot and two sets of toes. Much more. For a brief moment I wonder how much else about their lives, hidden behind the shiny façade, is also rotten and decayed. But then my professional demeanour returns. I become a barrier between them and the disease. I become crisp, efficient, businesslike. I make the telephone calls I have to make, say the soothing words that I have to say.

At the interface between the rotting chaos in the bed, and the obsessive neatness around me, I remain perfectly calm. I am a membrane, a barrier. I must be firm. But inside myself I am struggling to control those feelings and memories, the new smells mingling with the old, carrying me many thousands of miles away. Bad memories, another time, a different place.

Outside the quiet suburban street feels quite different to me. I am still thousands of miles away, somewhere hot and distant at the very bottom of Africa.

As a doctor you can never forget. Over the years you become a palimpsest of thousands of painful, shocking memories, old and new, and they remain with you for as long as you live. Just out of sight, but ready to burst out again at any moment.

Who can heal the wounded healer? The cancer specialist Rachel Naomi Remen has a novel suggestion. In her book *Kitchen Table Wisdom* she has written how sometimes doctors can be healed by their own patients, and not the other way round. She urges her colleagues to embrace the sense of uncertainty and ambiguity inherent in all clinical practice, and not to avoid it. To try to embrace their own vulnerability, and in this way be more open to their patients' humanity. And even, on occasion, to be open to being healed by them.

'One of the reasons that many physicians feel drained by their work,' she writes, 'is that they do not know how to make an opening to receive anything from their patients. The way we were trained, receiving is considered unprofessional. The way most of us were raised, receiving is considered a weakness.'

It's an inspiring prescription, but there is another way. To consider oneself as a type of secular shaman, a 'master of spirits', and, like them, to learn to overcome those dark feelings and moods within oneself, and all those horrifying memories, and then to use them for much better purposes.

So who then can heal the wounded healer? Only the healer himself. For, as Mircea Eliade has put it, in a remark that could as easily apply to many of the successful doctors I have known:

'The shaman is not only a sick man; he is above all, a sick man who has been cured, who has succeeded in curing himself.'

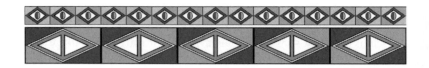

NOTES AND BIBLIOGRAPHY

Introduction

Page ix – The origin of the Osler quotation is: *Sir William Osler's Aphorisms From His Bedside Teachings and Writings*, collected by Robert Bennett Bean MD (Charles C Thomas, 1961). See Andrews BF. Sir William Osler's Emphasis on Physical Diagnosis and Listening to Symptoms. *Southern Medical Journal* 2002; 95(10): 1173-1177.

Page x – The quotation is from the Introduction to his *Cambridge Illustrated History of Medicine*, edited by Roy Porter. (Cambridge: Cambridge University Press, 1996, pages 6-15).

Page xi – Some of this background is described in my memoir: Cecil Helman *Suburban Shaman: Tales from Medicine's Frontline* (Hammersmith Press, 2006).

Page xiii – The excitement of the first heart transplant is well captured in Donald McRae's book *Every Second Counts* (London: Simon and Schuster, 2006).

Page xiv – A fuller version of the story of 'the man who turned black' is given in my memoir, *Suburban Shaman: Tales from Medicine's Frontline* (Hammersmith Press, 2006, pages 27-34).

Page xv – For more details on medical anthropology – the cross-cultural study of health, illness and medical care – see my textbook: Cecil G Helman. *Culture, Health and Illness*, 5th ed. (London: Hodder Arnold (now CRC Press), 2007).

Chapter 1: An Amazing Murmur of the Heart

Page 4 – Helman C (2006) *Suburban Shaman: Tales from Medicine's Frontline*, London: Hammersmith Press, Chapter 17: Grand Rounds, pages 127-133.

Page 7 – For a similar critical picture of American obstetrics, from an anthropological perspective: RE Davis-Floyd (1992) *Birth as an*

American Rite of Passage, Berkeley: University of California Press; and RE Davis-Floyd (1987) The technological model of birth. *Journal of American Folklore*, vol. 100, pages 479-495.

Page 9 – Gray H (1858) *Anatomy: Descriptive and Surgical*, illustrated by HV Carter MD, London: John W Parker and Son; Gray H (1909) *Anatomy: Descriptive and Applied*, 17th edition, London: Longmans, Green, and Co, and Standring S (editor-in-chief) *Gray's Anatomy*, 40th edition (2008) Elsevier, page 990.

Chapter 2: The Magic Machine

Page 10 – Grouse LD (1983) Editorial: Has the machine become the physician? *Journal of the American Medical Association*, vol, 259, page 1981.

Page 11 – The invention of new diagnostic equipment, from Laennec's stethoscope in 1816, to Roentgen's discovery of X-rays in 1895 and Herrick's invention of the electrocardiogram in 1918, all led to a greater ability to *localise* disease processes within the body. Sites of pathology could now be pinpointed with greater accuracy than ever before. It also meant that the body, not the patient's story, became the main medium for diagnosing disease.

Page 13 – An online description of the Visible Human Project (VHP) is: National Library of Medicine (2005) *The Visible Human Project*. http://www.nlm.nih.gov/pubs/factsheets/visible_human.html (Accessed 23 November 2006). The term 'computerized cadavers' was coined by Csordas, TJ (2000) Computerized cadavers. In: Brodwin PE (ed) *Biotechnology and Culture*. Indiana: Indiana University Press, pages 173-192.

Page 13 – The Human Genome Project (HGP) was an international project to 'map' the entire genome of the human organism. (The 'genome' of an organism is its entire genetic material, or DNA (deoxyribonucleic acid).) The project was completed in 2003 after 13 years' work, and at a cost of about US $3 billion. For more online information, see National Human Genome Research Institute (2006) *Genome* http://www.genome.gov/glossary.cfm?key=genome (Accessed on 25 March 2006). Also see Rheinberger H-J (2000) Beyond nature and culture: modes of reasoning in the age of molecular biology and medicine. In: Lock M, Young A, Cambrosio A (eds) *Living and Working With the*

New Medical Technologies, New York: Cambridge University Press, pages 19-30. 'Genetic determinism' means that the human organism is primarily 'a medium of communication and control', whose function is determined by 'genetically enshrined instruction'. For a strong critique of this see: Mauron A (2002) Genomic metaphysics, *Journal of Molecular Biology*, vol. 319, pages 957-962; and of this process in psychiatry: Kirmayer, LJ, Minas H. (2000) The future of cultural psychiatry: an international perspective. *Canadian Journal of Psychiatry*, vol. 45, pages 438-446. They warn of the limitations of the 'biologization' of the subject, and the view that brain dysfunction lies at the base of all psychiatric and behavioural disorders, while culture and other social factors are mere 'window dressing'.

Page 14 – Sandelowski M (2002) Visible human, vanishing bodies, and virtual nursing: complications of life, presence, place, and identity. *Advances in Nursing Science* vol. 24(3), pages 58-70. Turkle S (1984) *The Second Self: Computers and the human spirit*, London: Granada. See also her book on the internet, where she reaches similar conclusions: Turkle S (1997) *Life on the Screen: Identity in the Age of the Internet*, London: Simon and Schuster. The new sense of self-created by the internet has been called the 'cyber-self'.

Chapter 3: The *Dybbuk* of Eddie Barnett

Page 17 – An earlier version of this case was published as Helman C (1996) The Other Half of Eddie Barnett. *London Magazine*, vol. 36, Nos. 7 & 8, pages 29-38. All names and other identifying details in the case have been changed in order to protect the identity of the people concerned.

Page 21 – For a fuller description of *dybbuks* (also spelled '*dibbuks*') see Alan Unterman (1991) *Dictionary of Jewish Lore and Legend*, London: Thames and Hudson, pages 62-63; Jerome Trachtenberg (1970) *Jewish Magic and Superstition*, New York: Atheneum, pages 50-51; and Siegel R and Rheins C (eds) *The Jewish Almanac*, New York: Bantam Books, pages 334-336, 568-569, 596. For *dybbuks* in literature see Isaac Bashevis Singer (1974) The Dead Fiddler. In: *The Séance and Other Stories*, Harmondsworth: Penguin, pages 32-60, and (1958) *Satan in Goray*, Harmondsworth: Penguin Books. The first mention of a *dybbuk* was in 1571, though possession by evil spirits is also mentioned in the Bible (Samuel XVI:14, Samuel XVI:232 and Samuel XVIII:10). An introduction to Cabalistic thought is: Gershom GS (1969) *On the Kabbalah and its Symbolism.* New York: Schocken Books.

Page 22 – 'Spirit possession', especially in Africa and Europe, is covered in Lewis IM (1971) *Ecstatic Religion*, Harmondsworth: Penguin Books; Douglas M (ed) (1970) *Witchcraft Confessions and Accusations*, Tavistock; Mair L (1969) *Witchcraft.* World University Library; and Lewis-Williams D and Pearce D (2004) *San Spirituality.* Cape Town: Double Storey. Spirit possession in the Islamic world is described by Khalifa N and Hardie T (2005) Possession and *jinn, Journal of the Royal Society of Medicine* vol. 98, pages 351-353. In spirit possession, as with germs or viruses in the Western world, these pathogenic spirits are believed to reveal their identity by the particular symptoms that they cause, and can only be treated by driving them out of the body. In Western culture, a similar theme of 'possession' appears in movies such as *Invasion of the Body Snatchers* (1956) and *Stepford Wives* (1975 & 2004).

Page 22 – Briggs KM (1971) *A Dictionary of British Folk Tales.* Part B: Folk Legends, vol. 1, London: Routledge and Kegan Paul, pages 415-604. See also: Maria Leach (ed) (1972) *Funk and Wagnall's Standard Dictionary of Folklore, Mythology and Legends*, London: New English Library, pages 933-934; Thistleton Dyer TF (1893) *The Ghost World*, London: Ward & Downey/Philadelphia: J.B. Lippincott.

Page 24 – For a history of psychiatric 'electric shock therapy' see Porter R (2002) *Madness: A Brief History*, Oxford University Press.

Chapter 4: Stories like the Wind

Page 26 – An earlier version of this case was published as: Helman CG (1985) Disease and pseudo-disease: A case history of pseudo angina. In: Hahn RA, Gaines AD (eds) *Physicians of Western Medicine*, Dordrecht: Reidel, pages 293-331. All names and many other details in this case, as well as the one on page 32, have been changed to protect the identity of those concerned.

Page 26 – For a description of San beliefs and story-telling, see Skotnes P and Fleishman M (2002) *A Story is the Wind: Representing Time and Space in San narratives*, LLAREC/University of Cape Town; and

Lewis-Williams D and Pearce D (2004) *San Spirituality*. Cape Town: Double Storey. Descriptions of San exorcism are on page 91.

Page 30 – 'Cyberchondria' and other new 'internet diseases' are described in: Fisher R (2006) Just can't get enough: From cyberchondria to Google-stalking, technology is turning us into obsessive wrecks. *New Scientist*, vol. 192 (no. 2583/2584), pages 34-37.

Page 31 – Miller E (1998) The uses of culture in the making of AIDS neurosis in Japan. *Psychosomatic Medicine*, vol 60, pages 402-409. 'AIDS neurosis' is characterised by depressive symptoms, phobic tendencies and hypochondriacal thoughts. It may range from simple fears to delusional states and even suicidal tendencies; Miller D, Green J, Farmer R and Carroll G (1985) A 'pseudo-AIDS' syndrome following from fear of AIDS. *British Journal of Psychiatry*, vol. 146, pages 550–551.

Page 32 – Stokes W (1854) *The Diseases of the Heart and the Aorta*, Dublin: Hodges and Smith; Walshe WH (1862) *A Practical Treatise on the Diseases of the Heart and Great Vessels*, London: Walton and Maberly.

Page 32 – White PD (1951) *Heart Disease*. 4th edition. New York: Macmillan, (who called it 'false angina' or 'psychoneurotic chest pain'). Scott Peck M (1990) *People of the Lie*. New York: Arrow Books, page 136.

Page 33 – The term 'Munchausen syndrome' was first coined in 1931: Asher R. (1951) Munchausen's syndrome *Lancet*, vol. 1: pages 339-341. For descriptions of the syndrome, and some of its variants, see: Spiro HR (1968) Chronic factitious illness: Munchausen's syndrome, *Archives of General Psychiatry*, vol. 18, pages 569-579; and Park TA, Borsch MA, Dyer AR, Peiris AN (2004). Cardiopathia fantastica: the cardiac variant of Munchausen syndrome *Southern Medical Journal*, vol. 97(1), pages 48-52. This rare condition is characterised by clinical manifestations of acute cardiac disease that are feigned and recurrent, especially chest pain or breathlessness.

Page 33 – An example of *pseudologia fantastica* is: Snowdon J, Solomons R, Druce H (1978) Feigned bereavement: Twelve cases *British Journal of Psychiatry*, vol. 133, pages 15-19; Scott Peck M (1990) *People of the Lie*. New York: Arrow Books, page 136.

Chapter 5: Masks of Skin

Page 36 – The quotations come from: Stevens A, Lowe J (1997) *Human Histology* 2nd ed. London: Mosby, page 355; and Underwood JCE (ed) (2004) *General and Systemic Pathology*, 4th ed. Edinburgh: Churchill Livingston, page 675. In the case of 'Mary' I have changed her name and many other identifying details to protect her identity. The same applies to 'Janet'.

Page 40 – Benthien C (2002) *Skin: on the cultural border between self and the world*, translated by Thomas Dunlap. New York: Columbia University Press. Benson S (2000) Inscriptions on the self: Reflections on tattooing and piercing in contemporary Euro-America. In: Caplan J (ed) *Written on the Body*, [place]: Reaktion Books, pages 234-254.

Page 41 – For detailed ethnographic studies of tattooing, especially in the South Pacific (including Polynesia and Melanesia) see: Gell A (1993) *Wrapping in Images*, Oxford: Clarendon Press; and Hage P, Harary F, Milicic B (1996) Tattooing, gender and social stratification in Micro-Polynesia, *Journal of the Royal Anthropological Institute*, vol. 2, no 2, pages 335-350. For a history of tattooing in the West, also see Atkinson M (2003) *Tattooed: The sociogenesis of a body art*, Toronto: University of Toronto Press.

Page 42 – The discussion of 'boundary anxiety' is in: Marshall J (2004) The online body breaks out? Asence, ghosts, cyborgs, gender, polarity and politics *Fibreculture* Issue 3. http://journal.fibreculture.org/issue3/issue3_marshall.html (Accessed on 5 July 2005); McDougall J (1989) *Theatres of the Body*: Free Association Press.

Page 44 – For a discussion of the historical influences on Von Hagens's exhibition, including Vesalius, see: Cuir R (2006) Gunter von Hagens, inventor and imitator *Anthropology Today*, vol. 22, no. 6, pages 20-22.

Page 45 – For a discussion of Galenic models of the body, and the role of the skin, see: Smith V (2003) Better out than in. In: Boon T, Jones I (eds) *Treat Yourself: Health Consumers in a Medical Age*, London: Science Museum, pages 28-29. She describes how, because illness was believed to come from within, medical treatments aimed to 'draw out' the excess humours (blood, phlegm, black bile or yellow bile) from within the body, by various means including enemas and laxatives, inducing vomiting or sweating, massaging or bathing the body, or removing them via the skin – by 'sweating, blistering, poultices, cupping, bloodletting'. In modern psychotherapy, this may be the basis for the model of catharsis. Watts A (1973) *Psychotherapy East and West*, New York: Random House. For 'penetration' of the body by the 'medical gaze', see: Foucault M (2003) *The Birth of the Clinic*, London: Routledge, pages 107-130, 152-182.

Page 46 – Lawton G (2004) Extreme surgery *New Scientist*, vol. 184 (2471), pages 54-57; Falcon M (2000) Female genital surgery goes public. *USA Today Health*, March 3 2000. http://www.usatoday.com/life/health/doctor/lhdoc104.htm (Accessed on 14 October 2002).

Page 46 – For a discussion of the anthropological perspective on masks see Mack J (ed) (1994) *Masks: The Art of Expression*, London: British Museum Press. For a Jungian perspective on tribal masks, see Jaffé A 1968 (re-issued 2013) Symbolism in the Visual Arts. In: Jung CJ (ed) *Man and His Symbols*, New York: Dell Publishing, pages 257-322; and on psychological archetypes see: Jung CJ (1972) *Four Archetypes*, London: Routledge and Kegan Paul. See also: Eliade M (1986) *Symbols, the Sacred, and the Arts*, London: Crossroads Publishing Co, pages 64-71.

Chapter 6: Waiting for Godette

Page 49 – In the case of 'Jonathan' I have changed his name and many other identifying details, in order to protect his identity.

Page 49 – For a discussion of the anthropological view of myths, see: Seymour-Smith C (1986) *The Macmillan Dictionary of Anthropology*, London: Macmillan, pages 203-205. For a survey of creation myths see: Maclagan D (1977) *Creation Myths*, London: Thames and Hudson. See: Parrinder G (1967) *African Mythology*, London: Paul Hamlyn, pages 18-31 for descriptions of creation myths from many parts of Africa. The word 'myth' apparently stems from a root meaning 'utterance' (Maclagan, D *op. cit.* page 6).

Page 51 – The idea of 'personal myth' has some similarity to Eric Berne's concept of 'script' (Berne E (1978) *What Do You Say After You Say Hello?*, New York: Grove Press), but I am using 'myth' in the anthropological sense, where the story told and acted out usually includes more mystical, often religious or teleological elements.

Page 53 – For the Jungian perspective on myth, see: Maclagan D *op. cit.*, pages 5-10; and Jung CJ (ed) *Man and His Symbols*, New York: Dell

Publishing, pages 97-254. Byng-Hall J (1988) Scripts and legends in families and family therapy. *Family Process*, vol. 27, pages 167-79. He describes an inherited myth about his 18th-century ancestor Admiral Byng, that's played an influential role within his family for almost 200 years.

Page 56 – The quote is from Franz Kafka's story 'The Coming of the Messiah' (Das Kommen des Messias). In: *Parables and Paradoxes*, New York: Schocken Books, 1961, page 81.

Chapter 7: Healing and curing

Page 58 – 'Dr L' is a composite of several fine, humane doctors that I have been privileged to know, during my career. Medical anthropologists differentiate between the patient's perspective ('illness'), and that of the doctor ('disease'). *Illness* is the subjective response of an individual and of those around him to his being unwell; particularly how he and they interpret the origin and significance of this event; how it affects his behaviour and his relationship with other people; and the various steps he takes to remedy the situation. It not only includes his experience of ill health, but also the *meaning* he gives to that experience. *Disease* focuses mainly on observable and measurable changes in the body's structure or function, especially at the cellular, chemical or even molecular levels. '*Healing*' can be described as treating all the dimensions of 'illness' – physical, emotional, social and spiritual – while '*curing*' focuses mainly on treating the physical abnormalities of 'disease'. For more details see: Helman CG (2007) *Culture, Health and Illness* (5th edition), London: Hodder Arnold, pages 121-155. In: Cassell EJ (1976). *The Healer's Art: A New Approach to the Doctor–Patient Relationship*, New York: J. B. Lippincott, pages 47–83. Cassell uses the word 'illness' to represent 'what the patient feels when he goes to the doctor', and 'disease' for 'what he has on the way home from the doctor's office'. 'Disease, then, is something an organ has; illness is something a man has.'

Page 60 – For the effects of clock time and other forms of time on the human body and mind, see Helman CG (1987) Heart Disease and the Cultural Construction of Time: The Type A Behaviour Pattern as a Western Culture-Bound Syndrome, *Social Science and Medicine*, vol. 25, pages 969-979; Helman CG (2005) Cultural aspects of time and ageing, *EMBO Reports* (European Molecular Biology Organization), vol. 6 (Special Issue), pages S54-S58; and Hall ET (1984) *The Dance of Life: The Other Dimensions of Time*, New York: Anchor Press.

Page 64 – Benjamin Franklin's essay (1794) was reprinted in *Works of the late Doctor Benjamin Franklin*, London: Robinson, pages 60-65.

Chapter 8: The Psyche and the Soma

Page 68 – This paper is based on my published study: Helman CG (1985) Psyche, Soma and Society: The social construction of psychosomatic disorders, *Culture, Medicine and Psychiatry*, vol. 9, no 1, pages 1-26. The research was carried out at Harvard Medical School in 1983-84. Names, ages and other identifying details of individuals in the study have been changed to protect their identities.

Page 72 – Cassell EJ (1976) Disease as an 'it': concepts of disease revealed by patients' presentation of symptoms *Social Science and Medicine*, vol. 10, pages 143-146. The debate between the physiologists and the ontologists is described in Cassell EJ (1976) *The Healer's Art*, New York: J.B. Lippincott, pages 63-64. Ontological explanations include micro-organisms ('I picked up a germ', 'I've picked up a cold'), but they could also include other external agents such as spirits or *dybbuks*. Also see: Kaufman SR (1988) Towards a phenomenology of boundaries in medicine: chronic illness experience in the case of stroke *Medical Anthropology Quarterly* (New Series), vol. 2, pages 338–54.

Page 73 – Codell Carter K (1980) Germ theory, hysteria, and Freud's early work in psychopathology *Medical History*, vol. 24, pages 259-274. Before Freud, mental conditions such as hysteria were defined and classified by their symptoms, and not by their causes, and 'there were important similarities between the conception of hysteria in the 1880s and the conception of most diseases at the beginning of the century.'

Page 73 – Breuer J, Freud S (1966) On the Psychical Mechanism of Hysterical Phenomena: Preliminary Communication (1893) In: Freud S, Breuer J (1966) *Studies on Hysteria*, New York: Avon Books, pages 37-52. The 'abscess' model of psychopathology is in Freud's essay 'The Psychotherapy of Hysteria', pages 299-351. For descriptions of 'spirit possession', from an anthropological perspective, see page 68 (above).

Page 74 – For a history of the term 'psychosomatic', and a critique of the concept itself, see: Lipowski ZJ (1984) What does the word 'psychosomatic' really mean? A historical and semantic inquiry. *Psychosomatic Medicine*, vol. 46(2), pages 153-171. A fuller description of JCA Heinroth's work, including his *Textbook of Mental Disturbances* (1818) and other early work in psychosomatic medicine, is in: Porter R (2002) *Madness: A Brief History*, Oxford: Oxford University Press, pages 140-141. Examples of early psychosomatic theories of the reasons for 'organ choice', as well as 'personality' or 'character' theories of psychosomatic disorders, include: Bauer J (1942) *Constitution and Disease*, New York: Grune and Stratton; Sontag LW (1948) Determinants of predisposition to psychosomatic dysfunction and disease: Problem of proneness to psychosomatic disorder. In: Dunbar F (ed) *Synopsis of Psychosomatic Diagnosis and Treatment*. St Louis: CV Mosby and Co, pages 38-66; Weiss E, English OS (1942) *Psychosomatic Medicine*. Philadelphia: W.B. Saunders, pages 10-11; Dunbar F (1948) Introduction. In: *Synopsis of Psychosomatic Diagnosis and Treatment*, St Louis: CV Mosby and Co, pages 13-27; Gildea EF (1968) Special features of personality which are common to certain psychosomatic disorders *Psychosomatic Medicine*, vol. 11, pages 272-281; Knapp PH (1975) Psychosomatic aspects of bronchial asthma. In: Reiser MF (ed) *American Handbook of Psychiatry*, vol. 4 (2nd ed), New York: Basic Book, pages 693-707.
Page 75 – Cheren S, Knapp PH (1980) Gastrointestinal disorders. In: Kaplan MI, Freedman AM, Sadock BJ (eds) *Comprehensive Textbook of Psychiatry*, vol. 2 (3rd ed), Baltimore: Williams and Wilkins, pages 1862-1972.

Chapter 9: Double Deaths

Page 78 – Hertz R (1960) *Death and the Right Hand*: Cohen and West, pages 27-86. He points out that during the period between biological death and final social death, the deceased's soul is often considered to be in a state of limbo, still a partial member of society, and potentially dangerous to other people as it roams free and unburied. Perhaps this is why the families of the 'undead' in the Old Age Home are so reluctant to visit them. Descriptions of the 'double death' in different cultural groups are in: Eisenbruch M (1984) Cross-cultural aspects of bereavement. II: Ethnic and cultural variations in the development of bereavement practices. *Culture, Medicine and Psychiatry*, vol. 8, pages 315–47; Bryant CD (ed) (2003) *Handbook of Death and Dying* (2 volumes), London: Sage; Laungani P (1996) Death and bereavement in India and England: a comparative analysis. *Mortality* vol. 1(2), pages 191–212; and Suzuki H (2003) McFunerals: The transition of Japanese Funerary services. *Asian Anthropology* vol. 2, pages 49-78. In parts of rural India, widows were regarded as being 'socially dead' after the death of their husbands, and were expected to throw themselves onto his funeral pyre, sacrificing themselves in the ritual of *satee*. The practice has been illegal for many years.

Page 80 – The negative effect of belief (and of certain diagnostic labels) on mental and physical health is often called the *nocebo* effect (from the Latin *noceo*, 'I hurt'). For more details see: Hahn RA (1997) The nocebo phenomenon: concept, evidence, and implications for public health. *Preventive Medicine*, vol. 26, pages 607-611; and Helman CG (2001) Placebos and nocebos: the cultural construction of belief. In: Peters D (ed) *Understanding the Placebo Effect in Complementary Medicine*, Edinburgh: Churchill Livingstone, pages 3-16. A poignant and horrifying example of the negative effects of a doctor's attitudes and words on a patient's health is given in: Clark R (2002) *Upside Down and Inside Out*, Abingdon: Radcliffe Medical Press. This autobiographical piece was written just before she died from cancer. A similar picture is painted in Clive Sinclair's description of his kidney transplant, 'My Life as a Pig', from his book *A Soap Opera From Hell*, London: Picador, 1998. The figure of 'Lorraine' is based on an amalgam of several different individuals, with very similar experiences of medical treatment.

Page 82 – Engel G (1968) A life setting conductive to illness: the giving-up-given-up complex *Annals of Internal Medicine*, vol. 69, pages 293-300.

Page 82 – For an anthropological description of 'voodoo death' see: Lex BW (1977) Voodoo death: New thoughts on an old explanation. In: Landy D (ed) *Culture, Disease and Healing*, New York: Macmillan, pages 327-331. Something similar to voodoo death can occur in some religious or ethnic groups who emphasise marrying within that group, and who regard those 'marrying out' as socially dead, or at least as no longer full members of that group. In some communities, retirement or unemployment may have that same effect, especially among men. Levi-Strauss C (1967) *Structural Anthropology*, New York: Anchor Books, pages 161-162.

Page 83 – The story of 'Mrs P' and her family is not based on any individual person, or family. She is a composite of several different individuals, but with similar experiences of dementia.

Chapter 10: The Apotheosis of the Brain

Page 88 – The details on phrenology, and the work of Francis Joseph Gall (1758-1828) and Johann Caspar Spurzheim (1776-1832) are taken mainly from the entry on 'Phrenology' in the *Encyclopaedia Britannica*, 1910-1911 edition, vol. CCI, pages 534-541. Also the article by Steve Shapin, Homo Phrenologicus: Anthropological perspectives on an historical problem. In: Barnes B, Shapin S (1979) *Natural Order: Historical Studies of Scientific Culture*, London: Sage Publications, pages 41-66. On Spurzheim and Gall, also see: Porter R (2002) *Madness: A Brief History*. Oxford: Oxford University Press, pages 141-143. Gall, around 1800, originally called it 'cranioscopy' – 'a method to divine the personality and development of mental and moral faculties on the basis of the external shape of the skull' – and it was later renamed 'phrenology' by his follower Johan Spurzheim. In Britain their leading convert was George Combe, a lawyer in Edinburgh, and due largely to his influence scores of learned societies had been founded throughout the British Isles by the 1830s, dedicated to phrenology.

Page 89 – Much of this description of early anthropology, including the quote from AR Wallace, comes from the entry on 'Anthropology' in the *Encyclopaedia Britannica*, 9th edition, Edinburgh: Adam & Charles Black, 1875, pages 107-117. According to the same entry 'the conformation of the skull is second only to the colour of the skin as a criterion for the distinction of races.' There was much disagreement about how many races there actually were: a Professor Pickering described 11, Professor Bory St Vincent 15, while Professor Desmoulins claimed that there were no less than 16. As well as the 'Australoid', 'Negroid' and 'Mongoloid' races, most classifications included the Xanthrochroi (the 'fair whites') of north Europe and the Melanchroi ('dark whites') of southern Europe and the Celtic lands.

Charles Darwin's remark is quoted in: Miles R (1989) *The Woman's History of the World*, London: Paladin Books, page 227.

Page 89 – The Nazi institute was the headquarters of the *Deutsches Ahnenerbe – Studiengesellschaft für Geistesurgeschichte* (German Ancestry – Research and Teaching Society). It was founded by Heinrich Himmler, Hermann Wirth and Walter Darré in 1935, and incorporated into the SS in 1939.

Page 90 – See Frewin A (1974) *One Hundred Years of Science Fiction Illustration*, London: Jupiter Books, for many illustrations of these huge-headed 'extra-terrestrials', especially from the 1930s. Descriptions of over-cerebral 'super-villains' in comic books, such as 'Brain Wave', 'The Brain', 'Brainiac' and 'Brain Storm' are in *Who's Who: The Definitive Directory of the DC Universe 3* (1985) New York: DC Comics, and of the 'Mind Worm' in *Web of Spider-Man Annual*, (1967) vol. 1, no 1. New York: Marvel Comics. Several films, plays and stories have featured disembodied, autonomous heads: *Man Without a Body* (Eros Films, 1937), *Donovan's Brain* (Dowling Productions, 1953); Roald Dahl's story 'William and Mary' (in *Kiss, Kiss*, London: Penguin Books, 1969), and Samuel Beckett's play *Krapp's Last Tape* (1958).

Page 91 – For a contemporary description of the Decade of the Brain, and its aims, see: McAllister-Williams RH, Young AH (1990) The Decade of the Brain *Psychiatry in Practice*, vol. 9, no 3, pages 12-16. Details of US and Russian 'brain banks' are in Ascherson N (1991) Fallen idol. *Independent Magazine*, 16 November, pages 41–54. For details of 'brain banks' see: Diamond NL (1993) A brain is a terrible thing to waste, *OMNI*, August 1993, page 12.

Page 92 – The key text on establishing a definition of brain death was: Beecher HB, Adams RD, Berger AC, et al (1968) A definition of irreversible coma: a report of the ad hoc committee of the Harvard Medical School to examine the definition of brain death. *Journal of the American Medical Association*, vol. 205, pages 337–340. The first mention of a 'neomort' was in: Gaylin W (1974) Harvesting the dead – the potential for recycling human bodies, *Harper's Magazine*, September 28, vol. 249. The first country to adopt brain death as the definition of legal death was Finland in 1971. In 1980 the USA passed the Uniform Determination of Death Act (UDDA), which states that: 'An individual who has sustained either (1) irreversible cessation of circulatory and respiratory functions, or (2) irreversible cessation of all functions of the entire brain, including the brain stem, is dead. A determination of death must be made in accordance with accepted medical standards.' Diagnosis usually involves neurological examinations by at least two independent physicians. The UDDA definition was approved by the American Medical Association in 1980 and by the American Bar Association in 1981, and today all 50 states follow it as the legal standard of death. For transplantation issues in Japan, see: Nudeshima J (1991) Obstacles to brain death and organ transplantation in Japan. *Lancet*, vol. 338, pages 1063-1064, and: Aranami KY, Aranami Y et al (2000) Japanese Transplant law: a historical perspective. *Prog. Transplant* vol. 10(2), pages 106-108; and Japan Organ Transplant Homepage (2005) Current issues surrounding transplants and recipients http://www.jotnw.or.jp/english/08.html (Accessed on 10 August 2005).

Page 92 – Jonas H (1978) Against the stream: comments on the definition and redefinition of death. In: Beauchamp TL, Perlin S (eds) *Ethical Issues in Death and Dying*, New York: Prentice-Hall, pages 51-60.

Chapter 11: Heartsink

Page 96 – The seven 'heartsink' patients described here are not based on specific individuals. They are all composites, based on many different people, but all represent *types* of 'heartsink' patients that are commonly encountered in clinical practice.

Page 104 – Everitt SC, Birtwistle JH, Stevenson B (2002) *Oxford Handbook of General Practice*. Oxford: Oxford University Press, pages 868-869. The key text on 'heartsink' patients (also known as 'fat envelope' or 'fat file' patients) is Balint M (1964) *The Doctor, the Patient and the Illness* (2nd ed), London: Churchill Livingstone.

Page 106 – For a description of healing rituals, from an anthropological perspective, see my textbook: Helman CG (2007) *Culture, Health and Illness* (5th edition), London: Hodder Arnold, pages 224-244; Laderman C, Roseman M (eds) (1996) Introduction, In: *The Performance of Healing*, London: Routledge, pages 1-16: 'All medical encounters, no matter how mundane, are dramatic episodes. The protagonists, often without conscious thought, play out their respective roles of patient and healer according to their society's expectations.' And 'The power of the performance is a heightened intensity of communication, and enhancement of experience.' Also see Turner VW (1974) *The Ritual Process*, Harmondsworth: Penguin Books. Not all theatrical performances are healing, but most forms of healing involve some type of performance.

Page 107 – The inheritance of symptom patterns can be traced over several generations using a 'Family Health Tree': Prince-Embury S (1984). The family health tree: a form of identifying physical symptom patterns within the family. *Journal of Family Practice*, vol. 18, pages 75-81; or a 'genogram': Like R, Roger J, McGoldrick M (1988) Reading and interpreting genograms: A systematic approach *Journal of Family Practice*, vol. 26, no 4, pages 407-412, page 119. Much of this process, including the 'talk therapies', like psychotherapies, is what anthropologists term 'symbolic healing'. It involves the healer transforming the client's world-view, and emotional state, without necessarily curing their physical disease. It may take a religious or a secular form.

Chapter 12: Wounded Healers

Page 112 – Shem S (1978) *The House of God*, London: Black Swan. Also: Vaillant GE, Sobowale NC, MacArthur C (1972) Some psychological vulnerabilities of physicians *New England Journal of Medicine* vol. 287, no 8, pages 372-375.

Page 114 – Some of my own meetings with shamans are described in Helman C (2006) *Suburban Shaman: Tales from Medicine's Frontline*, London: Hammersmith Press, pages 159-170. For more anthropological descriptions of the shaman, and the process of becoming one – including their visions of fragmentation – see Vitebsky P (1995) *The Shaman*, London: Macmillan, pages 59-63. Descriptions of the shamanic practices and divinatory séances are in: Lewis IM (1971) *Ecstatic Religion*, London: Penguin Books, pages 37-38; and Halifax J (1979) *Shamanic Voices*, Harmondsworth: Penguin Books. She describes how becoming a shaman usually involves a major crisis, often an illness: 'an encounter with forces that decay and destroy. The shaman not only survives the ordeal of a debilitating sickness or accident but is healed in the process.' The shaman is thus 'a healer who has cured himself or herself; and as a healed healer, only he or she can truly know the territory of disease and death.' 'The shaman's ability to subdue, control, appease, and direct spirits separates him or her from ordinary individuals, who are victims of these powerful forces.'

Page 118 – The quote is from Remen RN (2000) *My Grandfather's Blessings: Stories that heal.* Riverhead Books. In his paper 'Sick doctors – ourselves' (*Update*, 1 May 1982, pages 1621-1627), the psychiatrist Glin Bennet also stressed the importance of doctors abandoning their authoritarian, omnipotent role, and admitting their own vulnerability and humanity when dealing with their patients. He also lists the health risks of being a doctor, including depression, suicide, alcoholism and drug abuse.

Page 119 – Eliade M (1989) *Shamanism: Archaic Techniques of Ecstasy.* London: Arkana.